Increase your Brainability—and Reduce your Risk of Dementia

Increase your Brainability—and Reduce your Risk of Dementia

CHARLES ALESSI

*Global Chief Clinical Officer, HIMSS; Senior Advisor,
Public Health England*

LARRY W. CHAMBERS

*Professor Emeritus, Department of Health Methods, Evidence and Impact,
Faculty of Health Sciences, McMaster University, Hamilton, Canada*

MUIR GRAY

Director of the Optimal Ageing Programme at Oxford

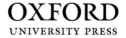

OXFORD
UNIVERSITY PRESS

OXFORD
UNIVERSITY PRESS

Great Clarendon Street, Oxford, OX2 6DP,
United Kingdom

Oxford University Press is a department of the University of Oxford.
It furthers the University's objective of excellence in research, scholarship,
and education by publishing worldwide. Oxford is a registered trade mark of
Oxford University Press in the UK and in certain other countries

First Edition published in 2021

Impression: 2

Published in the United States of America by Oxford University Press
198 Madison Avenue, New York, NY 10016, United States of America

British Library Cataloguing in Publication Data

Data available

Library of Congress Control Number: 2021932625

ISBN 978-0-19-886034-1

DOI: 10.1093/oso/9780198860341.001.0001

Printed and bound by
CPI Group (UK) Ltd, Croydon, CR0 4YY

Preface

We wrote this book to persuade readers to abandon negative and pessimistic beliefs about living longer because the science is clear that much of what happens to us is not the result of ageing, a normal biological process which cannot be slowed or reversed. Instead, science shows that many of the changes we have blamed on ageing are the result of other environmental factors which can be influenced. Furthermore, strong evidence from research has revealed many of these changes that were wrongly assumed to be the result of ageing can be prevented or delayed. We need to be positive, not negative, and being positive is also good for one's wellbeing.

People need this information, which in 2021 is of both vital and urgent importance, because the effects of lockdown have aggravated many of the problems that adversely affect physical and mental wellbeing.

This book was written for someone without a clinical qualification but many of our colleagues in our health systems are just as confused about ageing and dementia as members of the public and for them, as well as for the public we have provided references to the best science.

Our plan is to use this text as the platform for a major learning programme for people of all ages because, in the words of the Lancet which it used to launch the report of its Commission on Dementia, it is never too early and never too late to take action to increase the ability of the brain and reduce the risk of dementia.

Contents

Author Biographies

Former Scientific Advisor to the Alzheimer Society of Canada, Professor Chambers' research career has contributed to our understanding of many issues for people living with dementia. As a leader of the Canadian Study on Health and Aging, this was the first nation-wide Canadian population study of dementia prevalence, incidence, and caregiver issues by following the health trajectory of 10,000 older adult Canadians for 10 years. Professor Chambers co-led with the award-winning community wide program to prevent cardiovascular disease, a major cause of dementia. The Cardiovascular Health Awareness Program has received awards from the British Medical Journal, Canadian Institutes for Health Research, American Heart Association, and the Canadian Medical Association Journal. Professor Chambers' work on evaluating the effectiveness of community screening for the signs of dementia has received international recognition. With his colleagues, he has created E-learning education resources to promote interprofessional education with physicians, pharmacists, nurses, and nurse practitioners in care facilities, the main location of people living with advanced dementia in our communities. For these groups, he has created greater access to library services, establishment of a system-wide seniors' health knowledge network, as well as promotion of partnerships between academic and service delivery organizations such as care homes. Early in his career, Professor Chambers was an international scientific exchange fellow with the Research Unit on Neuropsychiatry: Epidemiology and Clinical Research, INSERM (medical research council), University of Montpellier, France. He has served on expert panels for Health Canada, US Institute of Medicine, WHO, and Pan American Health Organization. He has authored 18 books, 21 chapters in books, and 180 papers in refereed journals. Professor Chambers presently is Research Director of the Niagara Regional Campus, Michael G. DeGroote School of Medicine, McMaster University. He maintains appointments with the Department of Research Methods, Evidence, and Impact, McMaster University (Professor Emeritus); as well as with the Bruyère Research Institute., Faculty of Health at York University and IC/ES, Ontario's leading health and social data research organization. From 2013 to 2017, he was Scientific Advisor to the Alzheimer Society of Canada. He is a Fellow with the American College of Epidemiology, Honorary Fellow with the Faculty of Public Health of the United Kingdom and Fellow of the Canadian Academy of Health Sciences.

Muir Gray entered the Public Health Service in Oxford in 1972 after qualifying in medicine in Glasgow. He is a consultant in public health.

He has been working with both NHS England and Public Health England with the aim of increasing value for both populations and individuals and published *How To Get Better Value Healthcare* in 2007. The means of doing this through systems and personalization is now called population healthcare and the aim of population healthcare is to maximize value and equity by focusing not on institutions, specialties, or technologies, but on populations defined by a common symptom such as breathlessness, condition such as type 1 or type 2 Diabetes or by a common characteristic, such as multiple morbidity.

Recently he has returned to his first public health mission—preventing the changes we assume are due to ageing and disease by getting the right attitude and fighting back against an environment that makes us inactive. His key books include *Sod70!* And, with Diana Moran, *Sod Sitting, Get Moving!* He is the Director of the Optimal Ageing Programme at Oxford and its mission is to lead cultural revolution to change the way we think about living longer and this is now a national network involving all the key agencies with the manifesto and resources available at www. livelongerbetter.uk

Dr. Charles Alessi is a globally recognized and trusted leader in health care. He is the global chief clinical officer of HIMSS, a mission driven, not for profit global membership organization. He is a physician in London, with more than 35 years of experience in all aspects of clinical practice in the UK National Health Service. Most recently, he served as the Chairman of the National Association of Primary Care, part of the NHS confederation, where he was at the heart of the recent health and social care reforms.

He is also the Senior Advisor to Public Health England (PHE), a position leading thought leadership around productive healthy ageing including dementia, targeting risk reduction. Furthermore, he fulfils key roles in PHE around digital interventions, particularly those that involve behavioural change. Other responsibilities include air quality and antibiotic prescribing. He leads thought leadership around productive healthy aging. He has extensive experience in military medicine, being a past Medical Director and Director of Clinical Governance for the British Armed forces in Germany.

He holds a variety of international academic positions both in Europe and the Americas and has published widely in the media and journals. He is an Adjunct Research professor in Clinical Neurosciences at the Schulich School of Medicine at the University of Western Ontario, Canada and Visiting Scholar at the Odette School of business in Windsor, Ontario, Canada. He continues to advise major corporations and national governments around health and care reform, particularly where systemic reform and digital interventions are being considered.

1

Living Longer Better

Society has always had one disease that causes dread. In the first half of the twentieth century it was tuberculosis, or consumption as it was then known, a disease that was untreatable and which would slowly weaken and destroy the person before death. When tuberculosis became treatable, it became just another disease; of course it was better not to have it, but it had become something the medical profession could treat. Its place in our collective fears was taken by cancer. The 'big C', a disease, or to be more accurate several diseases, that evokes such fear that people are nervous of saying its name. Cancer continues to be a serious condition, but it is becoming a disease that is often curable, and almost always treatable. With the threat of cancer slowly diminishing, another disease is beginning to take its place as a source of dread: dementia, a condition that was hardly mentioned ten years ago, but is now regularly featured on the front pages of newspapers. The fear of dementia is complicated by the fear of ageing, and by muddled thinking about the relationship between the two. Before you become disheartened, it is important to emphasize that new scientific evidence means that we can be more positive and optimistic about the future.

As with tuberculosis and cancer, our thinking about dementia is changing, and scientists continue to search for an effective treatment for Alzheimer's disease and to increase the number of interventions that they can use to improve the quality of life of people with dementia, even if the basic cause of their dementia is the untreatable condition of Alzheimer's disease. For years, when people considered the future prospect of dementia, they would shudder and hope that, 'They'll have discovered a cure by the time I reach that age'. Although we can be optimistic that effective treatments will be developed, it would be foolish to do nothing in the meantime. No matter your age, the scientific evidence is clear:

Increase your Brainability—and Reduce your Risk of Dementia. Charles Alessi, Larry W. Chambers, and Muir Gray, Oxford University Press. © Oxford University Press 2021. DOI: 10.1093/oso/9780198860341.003.0001

- Your risk of dementia can be decreased.
- The capacity of your brain can be increased.

It may be that there will be no single treatment because Alzheimer's disease may prove to be several different conditions each of which will need its own specific treatment in the way that we now know that there are several breast cancers each with its own treatment.

Reducing your risk of dementia

This book has been written primarily for people who would like to reduce their risk of developing dementia; however, much of the information and advice we aim to provide, such as the need to prevent and decrease social isolation is still relevant to people who have already developed Alzheimer's disease or dementia.

There is no minimum age for people to begin thinking about reducing the risk of either Alzheimer's disease or dementia. It is now clear that factors occurring early in an individual's life course determine their risk of dementia. The results of a study undertaken in the USA showed that having a high school diploma is one of the most important differences between the people who did not develop dementia and those who did (Inouye, 2015).

Although people in their 20s, 30s, and 40s may think they are too busy, or too healthy, to worry about their future health status, there are two important factors to bear in mind.

- Many people in their 20s face considerable lifestyle challenges from such factors as employment in a job that requires a person to sit down for eight hours a day, together with a journey to work for an hour by train, bus, or car; inactivity, particularly if compounded by stress, is a major risk factor for dementia.
- Steps that can be taken to reduce the risk of dementia also reduce the risk of many other diseases, including:
  - Heart disease.
  - Stroke.
  - Cancers.
  - Type 2 diabetes.

If it is never too early to start reducing your risk of dementia, it is also never too late. The brain is not, as we once thought, an organ whose cells cannot divide and which start dying off from birth, but an organ with neuroplasticity, that is, the capacity to make new connections and build new networks that increase ability irrespective of age. The term 'neurogenesis' describes the creation of new functional units in the brain in adult life.

Thus, this book is relevant not only for people who are in their 40s, 50s, and 60s, but also for people in their 70s and beyond, for three reasons.

- There is no upper age limit for prevention.
- Steps for reducing the risk of dementia will also help you to reduce the risk of other diseases, to increase your fitness, and to feel better.
- If you have been told you have mild cognitive impairment (MCI) or dementia, or are concerned about someone who has been told this, all the measures we recommend for reducing the risk of dementia are also relevant for people who already have dementia. We now know that prevention and treatment are not two separate activities: after the onset of MCI or dementia, risk-reduction activities are equally as important as treatment.

Our current state of knowledge means that some causes of dementia cannot be prevented; there will always be an element of luck involved, but the decline in the number of people developing dementia in the last 20 years has been dramatic.

The shift from negative to positive

Things are changing, not because the elixir of life has been invented (although billions of dollars are being invested in this mission in the USA, with websites like Business insider predicting a market of over $38bn by 2024), but because we now understand more about the ageing process. We will describe this in more detail in Chapter 2, but in brief here:

- Ageing is not a cause of major problems until people reach the later 90s: look at David Attenborough, Her Majesty Queen Elizabeth II,

or John Goodenough, a winner of the Nobel Prize for chemistry in 2019, after being compulsorily retired from Oxford aged 65 years.
- The problems we fear—dementia, disability, and dependency—are due to three other processes:
  - Loss of physical fitness, which starts long before old age, for example, from when we obtain our first car or begin our first job where we sit for most of the time.
  - Diseases, whether preventable or not preventable, although you need luck to avoid those that are not preventable.
  - Negative beliefs and pessimistic attitudes.

Now we understand more about the ageing process, the following changes in society are taking place:

- A change from talking only about disability to talking about ability and how it can be improved at any age.
- A change from negative images and comments about people who are ageing to rejoicing in positive ageing; for instance, celebrating the achievements of Helena Jones, aged 101 years, who was given a British Empire Medal in the 2018 Honours list for 'services for young people and the community'.
- A change from bemoaning an inevitable loss of brain function to highlighting research that shows how the brain is resilient and can adapt and develop throughout life.
- A change from focusing only on dementia to a focus on Brainability.

This is not to say that Alzheimer's disease and dementia are not serious problems; they are. We now know, however, that much can be done to reduce the risk of dementia and improve Brainability even if dementia does develop.

In this book, we will focus on the positive, on how you can increase your Brainability. The good news is that everything we say about increasing Brainability will also reduce your risk of developing dementia. Everything you do to reduce your risk of dementia in the future will also reduce your risk of physical frailty and increase your Brainability in the here and now.

Our definitions—what do the terms 'dementia' and Alzheimer's disease really mean?

First, it is important to be clear about the meanings of terms we are going to use. When we started to conceive this book, we spoke to medical colleagues and found that many of them were just as confused as members of the public when trying to describe the relationship between dementia and Alzheimer's disease. Most of our colleagues who were not confused, however, were using these terms in different ways, almost all of them incorrectly.

If you consult the World Health Organization (WHO) *International Classification of Diseases,* dementia is defined as an 'organic mental disorder' (World Health Organization, 2018), namely, one caused by damage to the brain, as distinct from schizophrenia, which is a disorder of the mind. For diagnosis of dementia, the WHO requires evidence of:

- A decline in memory, which can be 'mild', 'moderate', or 'severe'.
- A decline in other cognitive abilities characterized by deterioration in judgement and thinking, such as planning, and organizing daily life; again, this deterioration can be graded as 'early stage', 'middle stage', or 'late stage'.

As the complete definition does not make for easy reading, our distilled definitions are shown in Box 1.1.

Other causes of dementia are a set of less common diseases, such as Pick's disease or Parkinson's disease.

The relationship between ageing and the brain

There is also some confusion about the relationship between ageing and the brain. The brain is affected by ageing like all other organs. As you live longer, changes take place in the brain. Dementia does not represent accelerated ageing. Ageing in any tissue or organ has two effects:

1. A loss of ability—for example even if Bradley Wiggins had continued to train, he would not have been able to improve upon the

Box 1.1 Distilled definitions of dementia, Alzheimer's disease, and vascular dementia

Dementia

Dementia is a condition that some people develop in old age, characterized by memory problems. Memory problems by themselves, however, are not a sign of dementia. The key issue is the impact of dementia on four functions:

1. The ability to manage financial affairs.
2. The ability to take care of your medical problems, such as taking the right pills at the correct time.
3. The ability to live safely without supervision.
4. The ability to drive a car safely.

The effect of dementia is determined by three factors:

- The severity of the dementia.
- An individual's personality before the dementia developed.
- An individual's social circumstances and support.

Alzheimer's disease

Alzheimer's disease is a disease of the brain of unknown cause; it is probably better described as several diseases with similar pathological changes and effects. Alzheimer's disease is one of the principal causes of dementia, but some people develop Alzheimer's disease without developing symptoms of dementia.

Vascular dementia

Vascular dementia results from impairment of the supply of oxygen-rich blood to the brain due to disease affecting the arteries within the brain. Many people have both Alzheimer's disease and vascular dementia, the relationship between these conditions is shown in Figure 1.1.

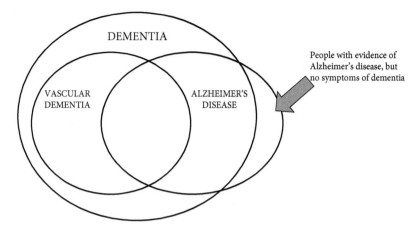

Figure 1.1 The relationship between dementia, Alzheimer's disease, and vascular dementia.
Copyright the Optimal Ageing Programme.

world record because the maximum rate at which the heart can beat decreases from 40 years of age.
2. A loss of resilience—resilience is the ability to bounce back after an injury, a disease, or a change in environmental temperature.

These two effects can be seen in what is referred to as 'cognitive ageing' and MCI. The American Alzheimer's Association and the Alzheimer's Societies of Canada and the UK define it as a disorder and the Canadian Society describes it in the following way: 'People with mild cognitive impairment (MCI) have problems with memory, language, thinking or judgement that are greater than the cognitive changes associated with normal aging' (Canevelli et al., 2016).

The Alzheimer's Society UK emphasizes that the benefit of diagnosing MCI is that the person can be helped to reduce the risk of developing dementia. A diagnosis of MCI does not mean that an individual will develop dementia, but that, in the words of the American Association, they are 'more likely to develop Alzheimer's or other dementias than people without MCI'. The Canadian Society points out that some people with MCI may improve.

The activities of the brain and mind are usually classified as being to do with emotion or to do with cognition, which is of greater concern. In normal cognitive ageing, the brain loses capacity to carry out activities

---

Box 1.2 Memory slips that the authors of this book experience frequently include recalling:

- The name of someone met yesterday.
- Where the car keys are.
- Where the mobile phone is in the house (ringing it while hoping it is not on silent).
- The author of a book that made a great impression when read twenty years ago.
- Whether one has double-locked the front door.

---

such as learning, problem-solving, quick decision-making, and remembering. Of these activities, a diminished capacity to remember is the most widely recognized and discussed. Many people worry that memory slips of the type listed in Box 1.2 are an early sign of dementia, but such slips do not mean that the development of dementia is inevitable.

Memory problems that should not be assumed to be signs of dementia

As mentioned earlier, another common sign of normal cognitive ageing is the loss of ability to make decisions quickly, for instance, when competing in a pub quiz. Although much is made of young people's superior decision-making speed, this is only one standard by which the quality of a decision should be judged. While one certainly needs quick decision-making when flying a fighter jet, many people do not need these skills; moreover, computers with artificial intelligence (the robots) are taking over many of the tasks that require rapid decision-making and hand/eye coordination (see Figure 1.2).

Furthermore, most decisions are not subject to intense time pressure, such as decisions about work and social life; indeed, it is possible to make such decisions too quickly. Oscar Wilde is credited with the following definition of experience as being, 'the name we give to our mistakes', highlighting the importance of experience. In general,

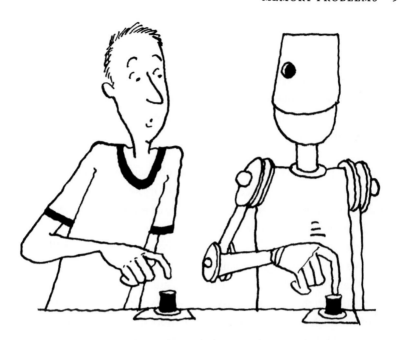

Figure 1.2 The fact that young people can make decisions quickly is no longer an advantage in the world of artificial intelligence.
Copyright the Optimal Ageing Programme.

older people have more experience, and are certainly no worse at making decisions that matter than young people. Older people may even be better at decision-making because they don't make decisions as quickly, having made many wrong decisions throughout the course of their lives.

In its report on cognitive ageing, the American College of Physicians, emphasized that although, 'some cognitive functions, such as memory and reaction time, decrease others such as wisdom and knowledge, increase with age' (Inouye, 2015).

People and publicity may focus on memory slips and decision speed because these aspects are noticeable and easy to measure, but neither of these changes are the cause of the types of problems people face because of dementia.

In a report on cognitive ageing by a group of notable dementia scientists convened by the National Academy of Sciences, Washington, DC (available free at www.nasonline.org), it is made clear that dementia becomes problematic when four key functions are affected:

- Looking after your financial affairs.
- Self-care and maintaining personal hygiene.
- Cleaning and maintaining a living space.
- Driving.

If these functions are affected, dementia represents a significant problem as opposed to the occurrence of minor memory slips, such as occasionally mislaying your keys or forgetting the name of someone you met last year.

It is important to appreciate the concept of brain reserve, and how it is affected by ageing. To understand the concept better, we will use the example of bone strength. If you should fall at 80 years of age, the probability that you will fracture your hip depends not only on how heavy the fall is, but also the strength of your bones. If your bones are thin due to a condition such as osteoporosis, you are more likely to sustain a fracture. The probability that you have osteoporosis is determined not by your diet or genes, but by how quickly you lose bone strength and how strong your bones were when you were at your prime. The decline in bone strength for two different people is shown in Figure 1.3.

From Figure 1.3, we can see that person A in early life was bigger and stronger than person B. However, although person A loses bone strength at the same rate as person B, person A does not develop osteoporosis because they have a greater reserve than person B. Person A is more resilient and can cope better with the demands not only of ageing but of an environment that offers little opportunity for people to continually challenge their bones, for example by carrying logs home to keep the fire burning. Similarly, some people have greater brain reserve, sometimes referred to as cognitive reserve, which means they have a greater level of resilience to cope with sudden demands or shocks. We can liken cognitive reserve to money in a bank account: the more there is to begin with, the easier is it to cope with unexpected large bills or financial demands.

For almost everyone, the actual rate of decline during normal ageing is faster than the best possible rate of decline, as shown in Figure 1.4. This is referred to as the 'fitness gap'. The good news is that the fitness gap can be closed at any age by increasing activity. The even better news is that the

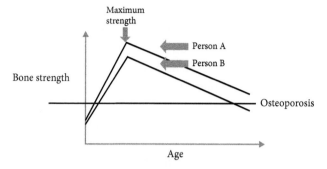

Figure 1.3 A comparison of the decline in bone strength in two different people showing that the level of strength at any age is determined, in part, by the maximum level before any decline starts.
Copyright the Optimal Ageing Programme.

fitness gap can be reduced even if the person has one or more long-term health problems.

This theory also applies to the brain. The higher the level of brain power you start with, the greater the brain or cognitive reserve, and the better you will be able to cope with any challenges to the way your brain

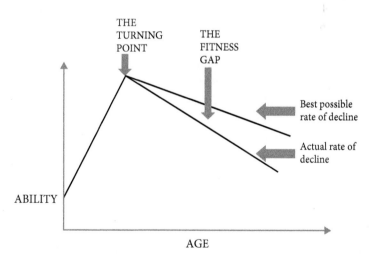

Figure 1.4 The fitness gap.
Copyright the Optimal Ageing Programme.

and mind work. Whether through increased isolation resulting from a disabling physical disease or the development of dementia the brain loses reserve, or witness to put it another way, if it becomes less active. The higher the level of brain or cognitive reserve you have, the longer you will be able to keep functioning without you or anyone else noticing any decline.

Naturally, it helps to start with a high level of Brainability but, as with bone strength, you can slow the decline and increase your cognitive or brain reserves at any age. Harvard Medical School has produced a commercial online programme called 'Cognitive Fitness'. The software includes clear information on the functions of the brain and on the training that can create new cells (neurogenesis) and new connections (neuroplasticity). The scientific understanding of what happens to the brain and mind as we live longer has increased significantly in the last twenty years and further reading is signposted in Box 1.3.

Box 1.3 Free high quality systematic reviews of the evidence

Blazer, D.G., Yaffe, K., & Liverman, C.T. (editors) (2015). Committee on the Public Health Dimensions of Cognitive Aging. Cognitive aging: Progress in understanding and opportunities for action. Board on Health Sciences Policy; Institute of Medicine. Washington, DC: National Academies Press. 21 July 2015.

Caamano-Isorna, F., Corral, M., Montes-Martinez, A., & Takkouche, B. (2006). Education and dementia: A meta-analytic study. *Neuroepidemiology*, 26(19), 226–232.

Canevelli, M., Grande, G., Lacorte, E., Quarchioni, E., Cesari, M., Mariani, C., et al. (2016). Spontaneous reversion of mild cognitive impairment to normal cognition: A systematic review of literature and meta-analysis. *Journal of the American MedicaAssociation*, 17(10), 943–948. doi: 10.1016/j.jamda.2016.06.020. Epub 5 Aug. 2016.

Livingston G., Sommerlad A., Bullard C., Banerjee S., Brayne C., Burns A., et al. (2020). The Lancet Commission on dementia prevention, intervention. *Lancet* 396, 413–416.

Finally, it is important to remember that once a diagnosis of dementia is made, the individual is still the person they were. It is important to be aware that the emotional and the cognitive aspects of the mind are not distinct in the way that the heart and the lungs are separate organs. Although the primary focus of dementia research is on the cognitive functions of the mind, there is growing interest in maintaining a person's well-being. The way people feel can increase their risk of dementia, and depression is now acknowledged to be a risk factor for dementia. Furthermore, if dementia develops, depression can often occur. We are interested in helping you feel better, as well as think better, but first you need to understand what is happening as you live longer.

References

Canevelli, M., Grande, G., Lacorte, E., Quarchioni, E., Cesari, M., Mariani, C., et al. (2016). Spontaneous reversion of mild cognitive impairment to normal cognition: A systematic review of literature and meta-analysis. *Journal of the American Medical Directors Association*, 17(10), 943–948. doi: 10.1016/j.jamda.2016.06.020. Epub 5 Aug. 2016.

Inouye, S.K. (2015). Enhanced cognitive aging: Clinical highlights of a report from the Institute of Medicine. *Annals of Internal Medicine*, 4, 307–310.

World Health Organization. (2018). The International Classification of Diseases and Related Health Problems 10th Revision.

2

Understanding the Potential
for Protecting
and Improving Brainability

This book has been organized to provide you with information and advice about how you can strengthen the ability of your brain and your mind. The same information and advice will also reduce your risk of dementia, but this book is about more than just dementia, hence its title is *Increase your Brainability*, with dementia in the subtitle.

When dealing with problems that affect older people the focus is almost always on negative topics, emphasizing disability and handicap. Obviously, it is vitally important for health services to focus on the treatment of disease and to minimize its disabling effect, but this often results in depression and low motivation for both the person affected and for their family and carers. The person affected may lose even more ability, developing a vicious cycle. Modern life is disabling because of the impact of the environment in which we live. However, a change is happening. Without losing our commitment to diagnose disease and treat disease effectively, the medical profession and the health service now recognize the need to provide care with empathy and a positive attitude.

In clinical psychology, the focus is now on an approach that is often termed positive psychology and this does not simply mean that a person should put on a Pollyanna smile, but that there is a need to recognize and try to change negative thoughts which dominate a person's thinking and then affect their ability. The aim of positive psychology is to help the person learn how to focus on positive thoughts. Increasing physical activity often helps too. For this reason, it is important to focus on the brain's ability and how it can be improved. All the steps you take to improve the

Increase your Brainability—and Reduce your Risk of Dementia. Charles Alessi, Larry W. Chambers, and Muir Gray,
Oxford University Press. © Oxford University Press 2021. DOI: 10.1093/oso/9780198860341.003.0002

ability of your brain will reduce the risk of dementia, but it is good to focus on the positive rather than the negative.

How preventable is dementia?

Over the last 20 years, there has been a decline in the proportion of people developing dementia of at least 20%. For example, a major study from Harvard, published in one of the world's most respected medical journals came to this conclusion:

'The five-year age- and sex-adjusted cumulative hazard rates for dementia were:

- 3.6 per 100 persons during the first epoch (late 1970s and early 1980s).
- 2.8 per 100 persons during the second epoch (late 1980s and early 1990s).
- 2.2 per 100 persons during the third epoch (late 1990s and early 2000s)
- 2.0 per 100 persons during the fourth epoch (late 2000s and early 2010s).'

We believe that further decline is possible.

Imagine that 1,000 people read this book and that 100 will develop dementia before they die. If our only objective was the prevention of dementia we would be delighted if only 70 developed dementia because that would be a 30% reduction in number of readers developing dementia. However, we are also interested in the 920 people who will not develop dementia. If even one half of them put into practice the advice in this book they would not only have reduced their risk of dementia, but they would also keep their brains healthier, their minds sharper, and:

- Develop fewer diseases.
- Be more able-bodied.
- Be more active and independent.
- Be less likely to have to go into a care home.
- Feel better.

But we don't want to give the impression that everything is preventable, that if something bad happens to you it is your fault, because that is not the case. Often books written to inform people about ways in which they can feel better and reduce their risk of disease simply cause guilt and depression. But there are two important principles that we wish to emphasize. The first is that many of the factors that affect your ability adversely and increase your risk are caused by the modern environment. The second is that you are not alone.

The modern environment causes modern epidemics

For thousands of years human beings evolved in a world in which there was little food, lots of activity, plenty of danger, and a short lifespan. The genes that favoured the ability to do without much food and run fast were favoured for millennia, but in the last two generations the environment has changed to one in which there is too much food and too little activity. Interestingly, although danger from sabre tooth tigers, and club wielding neighbours has declined, a new type of danger has developed: stress combined with inactivity. When danger required you to fight or flee, the stress reaction was helpful. However, when the danger must be faced when immobile, such as a boss breathing down your neck or an angry client across a table, you cannot fight or flee, and so the stress reaction causes inflammation.

The inflammation is not the red, tender inflammation that is an acute and healthy response to an infected cut, instead it is a silent, long-term inflammation which affects many tissues, including the brain. Scientists now think that this type of inflammation is a cause of many serious conditions. The problem is, in the words of the distinguished Harvard Professor Daniel Lieberman, that we still have Palaeolithic caveman bodies in what he calls a 'post Palaeolithic world' (Lieberman, 2014).

So, the problem it is not just ignorance or weakness, but a 'mismatch', to use Lieberman's term, between our genetic make-up and the environment in which we live. We are living longer, thanks to clean water and to better care for women in pregnancy and for children in the first few years of life, but new health problems are emerging—obesity, type 2 diabetes, and high blood pressure, to name but three. These problems result from an environment in which an increasing proportion of people must sit for eight hours a day, with another hour, still seated and commuting under stress, in a traffic jam, both before and after the day at a desk job. Palaeolithic men and women had many problems, but obesity and type 2 diabetes were not among them. Palaeolithic man's blood pressure occasionally went sky high as part of a stress reaction triggered when he and a fellow hunter encountered an angry tiger. But this change in pressure was temporary and lasted only as long as it was needed, which was until he outran either the tiger, or more likely, his fellow hunter, who would thus divert the tiger's attention for long enough for him to escape. The mismatch between our genes and the environment does not inevitably cause problems. We can adapt to the changed world in which we now live, either alone or working with others.

You are not alone

Obviously, you are on your own reading this book. Reading is a private activity, that is one of its pleasures, and it is very good for your mental health (Davis, 2020). However, that does not mean the authors of this book assumed that you would just close it and put the theory into practice the next day. That is not the way change happens and you need support from several sources which we will describe with respect to each risk factor.

First, there are family and friends. Research shows that their support is of crucial importance. If they, too, decide to change their behaviour then change is more likely, and friends include colleagues at work. Fortunately, employers and managers now understand that by encouraging healthy behaviour at work. With standing desks or ten minutes of brisk lunchtime walking, employers can help their employees improve their health and reduce their risk. They do this knowing that they will probably get more and better work from their employees, which will be a bonus for the company.

Second, there is support from the community in which you live. It has become fashionable to say that community spirit is non-existent. This is not the case. It is more difficult for community spirit to grow strong when there is a high rate of movement in and out of the village or estate.

However, in every community individuals emerge who are able to persuade people to work together and one strategy is to work with groups in the community, with 'old peoples clubs' or 'sports clubs', for example. These venues encourage members to put health on their agenda. There is another community, quickly developing, the online community, where people with similar interests can easily be put into contact. Parkrun is an excellent example of an organization of the Internet age that is enabling people to improve their health and have fun.

Third, there are people working for your health service and other professionals who can give information. This book falls into that category, with the information abbreviated to make it easily digestible. However, what is often needed is to speak with your doctor about any concerns. There are few reasons why someone with one, or more than one, long-term health problems should not follow all the advice in this book. If the authors had their way (and they plan to get it), everyone with a long-term health problem would be given the information in this book, and the support to put it into practice. Modern drugs are wonderful for conditions like heart failure, type 1 diabetes, and Parkinson's disease, but drug therapy alone is not what benefits most. Of course, it is not just health service professionals who can provide support. Trainers working in gyms, fitness clubs, and wellness centres are also trained to support people with long-term health problems, in addition to pushing the Lycra wearing youngsters into sweating more. There are plenty of people keen to help.

Though some research (Peters et al., 2019) has shown a link between living near a highway and several neurological diseases, the evidence is not strong enough at present to draw a strong conclusion. The condition of the world we live in is determined to a large extent by big business and politics. Although politics can be easier to influence than big business, more support from government, both national and local is needed to combat the effects of modernization. The modern city is designed with cars as a central pivot, not the citizens who prefer to walk or cycle. Perhaps the most important thing that politicians can do in the long term is to ensure that every child gets a good education and is brought up in a society that values education. Because a poor childhood education and all that this entails, seems to be as important a risk factor as those that can be identified and reduced from middle age on. One important point is that getting involved politically, which includes, arguing, reflecting, attacking, and being attacked is one of the best activities for maintaining and improving mental ability and therefore reducing the risk of dementia.

Advice based on evidence and experience

'Rhubarb prevents dementia' is a headline we have never seen but would not be surprised if it appeared on the front page of a newspaper. Nor would we be surprised by a headline 'Rhubarb cures dementia'. Neither headline would make us change what we do immediately because headlines like that are usually based on the report of a single research project and single studies are unreliable. One of the key principles which we believe, and all other people who take an evidence-based approach to health and healthcare, is that you should never rely on a single research project, no matter how big it is. The evidence on which this book is based, is what is called systematic reviews of the evidence. To prepare a systematic review, the researcher must:

- Identify all the research done on a topic.
- Classify all the studies as being either reliable or unreliable.
- Combine all the results of the reliable studies into a single result.

All the advice in this book is based on systematic reviews or, what are sometimes called 'umbrella reviews' of all the systematic reviews that have been done about a topic. There are often different research groups taking a slightly different perspective on the benefits of physical activity among other things. This work is led by an organization called the Cochrane Collaboration whose mission is to promote evidence-informed health decision-making through producing high-quality, relevant, accessible systematic reviews and other synthesized research evidence.

The *Lancet* medical journal published a systematic review in 2017, which is available free on their website. The details from this report and other key studies are listed in Box 2.1.

Based on our own experience and high-quality systematic reviews of the evidence (Box 2.1), we have identified several steps that you can take to increase your ability. It is unlikely that a pill that reduces your risk of Alzheimer's disease will be created in the next few years. So, we have

Box 2.1 Free high-quality systematic reviews of the evidence

Anstey, K.J., Ee, N., & Eramudugolla, R. (2019). A systematic review of meta-analyses that evaluate risk factors for dementia to evaluate the quantity, quality, and global representativeness of evidence. *Journal of Alzheimer's Disease* 70(s1): 1–21. doi: 10.3233/JAD-190181.

Blazer, D.G., et al. (2017). *Cognitive Aging: Progress in Understanding and Opportunities for Action, Institute of Medicine*. National Academy of Sciences.

Global Council on Brain Health (2015). *Engage Your Brain: GCBH Recommendations on Cognitively Stimulating Activities*. Washington D.C.: American Association of Retired Persons.

Lafortune, L., Kelly S., Olanrewaju O., Cowan A., and Brayne C. (2016). *Changing Risk Behaviours and Promoting Cognitive Health in Older Adults: An Evidence-Based Resource for Local Authorities and Commissioners*. Prepared by the Cambridge Institute of Public Health, University of Cambridge Public Health England.

Leshner, A.L. (2017). *Preventing Cognitive Decline and Dementia; a Way Forward Committee on Preventing Dementia and Cognitive Impairment; Institute of Medicine.*; National Academy of Sciences.

Livingston, G., Sommerlad A., Orgeta V., Costa Freda S.G., Huntley J., Ames D., et al. (2017). The Lancet Commission on 'Dementia prevention, intervention, and care'. *Lancet*, 390, 2673–2734.

NICE (2015). *Dementia, Disability and Frailty in Later Life—Mid-Life Approaches to Delay or Prevent Onset*. National Institute for Health and Clinical Excellence, London.

WHO (2015). *Ageing and Health*. World Health Organization, Geneva.

Tucker K. (2019). The New Science of Healthy Aging. Scientific American.

Alzheimer's Disease International (2014). Dementia and Risk Reduction.

Also consult the Harvard Medical School special health reports, written for the public but of high quality, for example: *Improving Memory, Understanding Age-Related Memory Loss*. www.health.harvard.edu Boston.

identified three strategies for the person who wants to increase their brain ability to follow. We call it our Triple Whammy Brainability Programme:

- Keep your brain tissue healthy.
- Keep the blood supply to your brain flowing well through healthy arteries.
- Stay engaged or get more engaged and involved with other people.

These three things will be further explored in the next three chapters of the book. Though this suggests that they are three separate strategies, they in fact overlap and interrelate. For example:

- Increasing your physical fitness is not only good for your arteries, but it also has a direct effect on the brain tissue and, by keeping you mobile, helps you keep engaged with other people.
- Managing stress better helps you sleep better and feel better and this makes it easier to focus on enjoying the company of other people and on changing your diet to keep your arteries healthy.

So, it is helpful to present the contents of the remainder of the book not as a list but as pictures, such as the Venn diagram shown in Figures 2.1–2.5. Another way of emphasizing the interconnectedness is to show them not as a list but as three activities, each of which interacts with the other two.

'What the hell is happening to me?'

Let's be clear about what is happening to us as we live longer, because most people are confused. Four things are happening:

- Everyone is affected by ageing, but ageing by itself is not a cause of major problems till the later 90s, if ever. Some centenarians are clear as a bell.
- Most people are affected by loss of fitness, physical, mental, and social:
  - Physical fitness is lost because of the environment we live in.

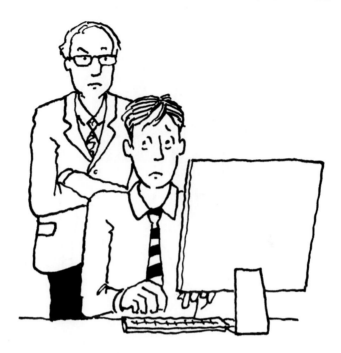

Figure 2.1 Modern stress combined with inactivity.
Source the Optimal Ageing Programme.

- Mental or cognitive fitness is lost if we are not engaging our brain in challenging problems.
- Social or emotional fitness is lost if we interact less with others and, for many people, isolation caused or complicated by problems with hearing and seeing, leads to significant loss of function.
- Some people are affected by the diseases that cause dementia, the most common being Alzheimer's and diseases of the blood supply to the brain, which often occur together.
- Almost everyone has incorrect negative beliefs about what happens as we live longer.

So, we need a new approach, we need to understand and accept ageing, get fitter, reduce the impact of disease, and think more positively.

So, let's act.

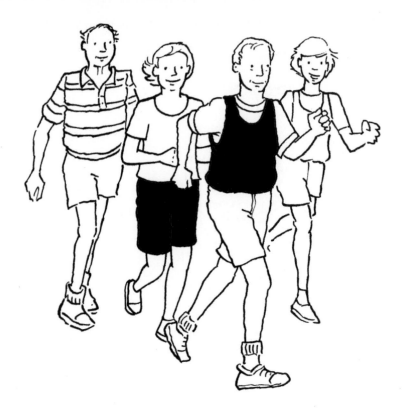

Figure 2.2 Parkway running is a new health service.
Source the Optimal Ageing Programme.

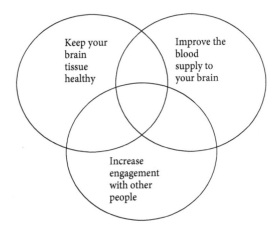

Keep your
brain
tissue
healthy

Improve the
blood
supply to
your brain

Increase
engagement
with other
people

Figure 2.3 The three strategies to increase Brainability and reduce the risk
of dementia overlap.
Source the Optimal Ageing Programme.

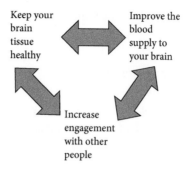

Figure 2.4 The three factors enhance and interact with the other two.
Source the Optimal Ageing Programme.

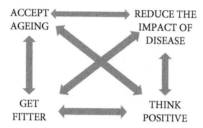

Figure 2.5 The four processes that affect ability and well-being.
Source the Optimal Ageing Programme.

The Triple Whammy Brainability Programme

Based on this way of looking at living longer we have developed the Triple Whammy Brainability Programme, which has three strands of equal importance and set out below are the sections and subsections of the book.

Keep your brain tissue healthy:

- Get more active and physically fitter.
- Reduce the impact of stress.
- Sleep better.
- Be wary of over medication.

Increase the blood supply to the brain:

- Stop smoking.
- Keep your blood pressure low.
- Keep your weight down.
- Find out if you have atrial fibrillation and get it treated.
- If you have had a transient ischaemic attack (TIA), act.
- Rebalance your diet through keeping your sugar intake and cholesterol low.

Increase the ability of your mind to interact with people and ideas

- Get even more active and involved to minimize isolation and depression.
- Increase intellectual activity.
- Check your hearing and vision.

We start with keeping your brain tissue healthy.

References

Davis, P. (2020). *Reading for Life*. Oxford: Oxford University Press.

Lieberman, D.E. (2014). *Alcohol and Dementia. The Story of The Human Body: Evolution, Health, and Disease*. London: Penguin.

Peters, R.E., Nicole E., Peters J., Booth A., Mudway I., Anstey K.J. (2019). Air pollution and dementia: A systematic review. *Journal of Alzheimer's Disease*, 70: s1: S145–S163.

3

Keep Your Brain Tissue Healthy

The body needs protection from damage. The environment we live in is full of threats to our bodies, threats from our environment and the lives we lead, and the brain needs protection from harm. There is growing concern about the damage caused not only by boxing but also by rugby and football. Concerns about the possibility that environmental pollution also damages the brain are also steadily growing. Some research has shown a higher rate of dementia among people who live near busy highways. Diesel doesn't represent the only threat, as many other chemicals and microscopic particles are produced by cars. But the ever-present danger to human health of the effects of pollution, if proven, will not compare with the single major health threat from cars—inactivity.

The main threats to brain tissue are internal, and can be countered by four steps:

- Reduce the impact of stress.
- Sleep better.
- Be wary of over medication.
- Get more active and physically fitter.

Reducing the impact of stress

Coping better with stress and dealing with the causes of stress help you feel better immediately and reduce the risk of dementia.

Acute stress increases your heart rate, your lungs take in more oxygen, your blood flow increases, and parts of your immune system become temporarily suppressed, reducing your body's inflammatory response to pathogens and other foreign invaders. By managing acute

Increase your Brainability—and Reduce your Risk of Dementia. Charles Alessi, Larry W. Chambers, and Muir Gray, Oxford University Press. © Oxford University Press 2021. DOI: 10.1093/oso/9780198860341.003.0003

stress, your body will not release stress hormones such as cortisol that prepare your body to either fight or flee the stressful event. When stress becomes long term, your immune system becomes less sensitive to cortisol, and since inflammation is partly regulated by this hormone, this decreased sensitivity heightens the inflammatory response and allows inflammation to get out of control. Long-term inflammation, in turn, is a hallmark of most diseases, from diabetes to heart disease, cancer, and dementia. You can reduce your stress yourself through a variety of methods, including physical activity and mindfulness. Also, friends and family can be helpful, or seeking out your doctor to put you in touch with a psychologist who employs what is called cognitive training. This involves helping you learn patterns of thinking that are positive, and which give you the feeling of control that reduces stress.

What is meant by stress management?

It is common to think of stress as one of the plagues of modern life, and dream of living in stress free environments where there is no pressure to perform or deadlines to manage. We imagine living our lives lounging on a sunbed under an umbrella all day with a cold drink on our left and a vista of swaying palm trees on our right. Reality is somewhat different because some stress, manageable stress, should be viewed as stimulating and beneficial, as well as health promoting. We know of the benefits of physical stress, achieved through physical exertion, which need to stretch us and make us sweat a little for it to be truly beneficial. The same analogy applies to mental stress, where we need a little pressure to keep us truly engaged and involved. Thus, the emphasis should be on managing unnecessary and excessive stress, not removing stress completely.

Stress shouldn't always be viewed as something negative. Figure 3.1 shows stress measurements in relation to performance, which highlights that optimal performance needs to be accompanied by manageable levels of stress. Once levels of stress increase and become adverse it is clear how performance suffers, with exhaustion and ill health to follow.

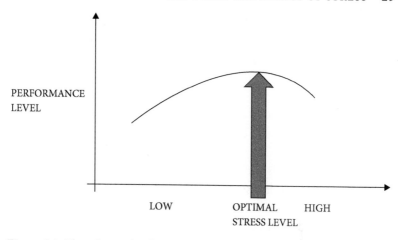

Figure 3.1 The relationship between stress levels and performance.
Source the Optimal Ageing Programme.

What is the risk of high stress? How common is it?

Stress is not an illness, but adverse stress is the feeling of being under too much mental or emotional pressure, which turns into stress when you feel unable to cope. A manageable level of stress is normal and can be beneficial by helping push you to do something new or difficult. Low levels of stress may result in poor performance and everyone from top level athletes to people in busy jobs know that feeling when you are just a bit on edge and nervous; for optimal performance the right level of stress is needed as shown in Figure 3.1.

When stress becomes too great, performance starts to deteriorate, and the person may become burned out. Should it become unmanageable, it can affect you adversely. It does so by taking its toll on your body and your immune system. Getting stress under control can boost your immune system and help prevent serious health problems, such as high blood pressure, heart disease, stroke, and dementia. Adverse levels of stress can also lead to disturbed sleep patterns, which in turn also predispose to heart disease and type 2 diabetes.

Stress can also affect how you feel and how you react to people. Learning how to manage stress can help you build and maintain positive relationships with those around you. We now know how important it is to avoid social isolation and avoiding adverse stress helps us maintain relationships. Adverse stress can also lead to chronic depression that is another of the risk factors for dementia.

How strong is the evidence about managing adverse stress in avoiding dementia?

There are several trials and systematic reviews looking at the association between chronic adverse stress and dementia. The factors that are deleterious to the heart are the same for the brain. The ageing brain has increased susceptibility to chronic stress and may also accelerate cognitive decline and dementia. The contribution of other effects of adverse stress on the heart and arteries and its effects on diabetes are also additive because this affects the flow of oxygen rich blood to the brain. These factors together make adverse stress something we need to avoid and manage.

So how does stress cause heart disease and diseases of the arteries? Stress is an integral part of being alive and a natural response to danger. At its most basic, the 'fight or flight response' is basically a response to potentially dangerous situations. In these situations, the body produces increased levels of the 'stress hormones' like adrenaline and cortisol, which help the body get ready to react even faster than normal. This is a wholly physiological and healthy response and does us no harm. Indeed, it is positively beneficial as it aids us in fleeing dangerous situations, like running away from danger faster. Stress becomes harmful when it is prolonged and persistent, and in these situations, chronic stress exposes your body to unhealthy, persistently elevated levels of stress hormones like adrenaline and cortisol. These high levels of hormones increase the risk of narrowing of the arteries in the heart and brain.

What appears to be one mechanism by which stress causes harm to the brain is when it occurs with inactivity. The fight or flight stress reaction was useful for cavemen living in the Palaeolithic era, when the fight or flight reaction helped them fight a sabre-toothed tiger, or, preferably run away from it (or simply faster than the other cavemen). However, the effect of the stress reaction when we are inactive, on the phone to a difficult client, or being criticised by our manager when stuck at our desk, leads not to fight or flight but to inflammation of the tissue of the brain.

Box 3.1 Free high-quality systematic reviews of the evidence

- Becker, E., et al. (2018). Anxiety as a risk factor of Alzheimer's disease and vascular dementia. *British Journal of Psychiatry*, 213, 654–660.
- Gulpers, B., et al. (2016). Anxiety as a predictor for cognitive decline and dementia: A systematic review and meta-analysis. *American Journal of Geriatric Psychiatry*, 24, 823–842.

We also know that adverse stress causes anxiety, affecting sleep, and poor sleep patterns are often the result. These in turn lead to an altered hormone balance that can affect food intake and weight. A lack of sleep also increases your risk of obesity and being obese can increase your risk of developing type 2 diabetes, a condition that also increases the risk of dementia. Stress also increases anxiety, which adds to the risk of dementia (Becker et al., 2018). There are thus many reasons why adverse stress is not good for us and we need to manage levels of stress to ensure we manage the risks of dementia better (see Box 3.1).

Am I on the right track in managing stress?

Managing adverse stress is something we all do. We do this all the time, but sometimes the levels of stress stay high for a long period of time and then we need to manage this differently (see Figure 3.2).

Many techniques exist to avoid stress—audio and video, games, apps and guides, and other tools. However, there are certain even more simple steps which everyone should adopt. These are:

- Start to think more about time management. Split your day into chunks, take regular breaks, and take a lunch break with a brisk walk to ensure you get a change of scene.
- Make lists of what you need to do and prioritize them in order of importance. Work out your goals and focus on the results you wish to achieve.

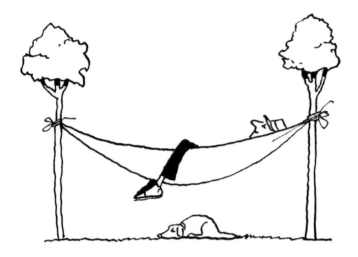

Figure 3.2 Many techniques exist to avoid stress.
Source the Optimal Ageing Programme.

- Take regular exercise, because the fitter you feel physically, the better you can function intellectually. Choose to use a bus stop or parking lot a little further from your work and try to ensure you walk more often. It also helps you socialize and feel part of the wider world. Walking in or near forests and woods is particularly helpful; in Japan what is called forest bathing is prescribed by doctors and cities try to maintain or create little bits of woodland even in the busiest cities.

Taking deep, soothing breaths when you are under stress can be helpful. Calming prayers or meditation can help you relax; the new term is 'mindfulness' which means becoming more aware of ourselves, our actions and their effects, and the environment we inhabit. It sounds self-evident, and it is, but sadly many of us lead too rushed a life to notice where we are and what is going on around us. There are simple techniques we can use to manage this better; the techniques involve training in observing, acknowledging, and accepting thoughts and feelings. This approach can help manage stressful thoughts that cause emotional upset and flight-or-fight responses. Mindfulness based stress reduction (MBSR) therapy is a meditation therapy. Though originally designed for stress management it is being used for treating a variety of illnesses, such as depression, anxiety, chronic pain, cancer, diabetes mellitus, hypertension, and skin and immune disorders.

Resilience is our ability to manage adverse events like stress better. The more resilience we have the more reserves we have to help manage stressful situations. Some people find it easier to recover after having been through difficult times and these are the more resilient people. Some of us have learned to be more resilient through our childhood and experiences, but we can all learn how to become even more resilient by using simple behavioural modification techniques (see Box 3.2).

Box 3.2 Free high-quality systematic reviews of the evidence

Adam, P., et al. (2014). Impact of sleep on the risk of cognitive decline and dementia. *Current Opinions in Psychiatry*, 27(6), 478–483. doi: 10.1097/YCO.0000000000000106.

de Almondes, K.M., et al. (2016). Insomnia and risk of dementia in older adults: Systematic review and meta-analysis. *Journal of Psychiatric Research*, 77, 109–115.

Bubu, O.M., et al. (2017). Sleep, cognitive impairment, and Alzheimer's disease: A systematic review and meta-analysis. *Sleep*, 40, 1: http://dx.doi.org/10.1093/sleep/zsw032

Global Council on Brain Health (2016). The Brain-Sleep Connection: GCBH Recommendations on Sleep and Brain Health. Available at: www.GlobalCouncilOnBrainHealth.org. doi: https://doi.org/10.26419/pia.00014.001

Kim, H.B., et al. (2016). Longer duration of sleep and risk of cognitive decline: A meta-analysis of observational studies. *Neuroepidemiology*, 47, 171–180.

What sources of support are there for people who want to improve their management of stress?

In friends and family

Whichever stratagem we employ to better manage adverse stress, we are not alone. All of us are subject to stressful situations and all of us occasionally find the pressure too much to bear. Now you have better understood how this happens and what to do if stress is unduly prolonged and you feel you are developing chronic adverse stress, you have many tools you can use to manage this and reduce your risks. Friends and family can support you on many fronts. For example, listening to you and working with you to find ways to reduce stress. They can also assist you in locating resources to assist you in managing your stress in the community and in the health service.

In the community

In the UK, Canada, and the USA, a range of organizations provide support to people experiencing acute and long-term stress. For example, the UK Support Line suggests 13 ways you yourself can reduce stress. The Canadian government also has a stress management site.

In the health service

When looking at continuing problems around job pressures, relationship problems, or other life circumstances, counselling may help manage your stress. Also, you can ask your doctor about cognitive training which is more focused on how you think about the problems that are causing stress and how to deal with them better. The National Academy of Sciences review: *Preventing Cognitive Decline and Dementia: A Way Forward* (Becker et al., 2018) found cognitive training (interventions, including ones aimed at enhancing reasoning, memory, and processing speed) delayed slow age-related cognitive decline. It can be good for such difficulties as it focuses on helping you 'reframe' your thoughts, beliefs, and attitudes about your concerns. Changing the way you think, can change the way you feel. Cognitive training is available on a time-limited basis. People learn skills they can use to handle stressful situations. Counsellors can also provide tools to help you talk through conflicts with family or friends (see Box 3.3).

Box 3.3 The problem with pharmaceuticals

In a 2017 issue of the Canadian magazine *Zoomer*, journalist, Sally Armstrong, reported on: 'Betty, 86, the poster girl in Canada for polypharmacy whose story is a cautionary tale in aging and doctor care. Luckily for Canadians, Betty, a high-energy, fun-loving senior, took her story to CBC's *Go Public*.'

Here is the frightful story she told. 'It started with an ear infection. I was given an antibiotic to clear it up. Pretty soon, I had painful swollen legs. I had cataract surgery two weeks later. I was given the drug prednisolone.' Three weeks after that, she was given another drug for ongoing pain in her ear. Then, she also used ibuprofen to deal with the pain in her leg and her ear. The polypharmacy cycle had begun. Betty went to her doctor and told him about health issues she had never experienced before. 'I was confused. The noises in my head sounded like Niagara Falls. My Achilles tendon was painful and swollen. I was acting in ways I never acted before, being outspoken and saying things I wouldn't normally say.' Without explaining what he was doing, the doctor administered a cognitive test to Betty. She failed it. He declared her incompetent and had her driver's licence revoked. 'I was sick that day. I was running a fever, feeling terrible. What's more, I read lips because my hearing is not what it used to be, and he was looking at a screen asking me questions that I couldn't hear or understand. I went to the doctor to ask for help. And this is what I got.' Betty was furious. 'I knew I was not incompetent and decided I was going to get to the bottom of what had happened to me myself.' She started by googling the names of the drugs she was on and almost immediately diagnosed her own problem. She met with a new doctor, who agreed that her symptoms were a result of the drug reactions. She stopped taking them and 'in a matter of about 10 days, I was fine'. This is precisely what happens when certain drugs are mixed and given to older adults. 'Side effects include confusion, memory loss and aggression—symptoms that may be misdiagnosed as dementia.'

'It cost Betty to undo what the doctor did. She had to pay a fee to take another cognitive test and prove she was of sound mind and another fee to take a new driving test to get her licence back. She passed both. But the humiliation she felt, the out-of-pocket costs to get to a town where she could have the tests and the anxiety that resulted were additional expenses that Betty does not forget.'

Sleep more and sleep better

Adequate sleep is a major factor that can improve cognitive abilities and reduce the risk of dementia. Adequate sleep is important for everyday good health. Too little sleep (less than six hours), or too much (more than nine hours), is associated with reductions in cognitive ability. Ways to prevent or control insomnia include:

- Getting regular exercise.
- Avoiding high calorie snacks, sugar, large amounts of caffeine, and extreme levels of activity late in the evening before going to bed.

Methods that help to gain a restful sleep include:

- Having a quiet, cool bedroom with little or no light.
- Taking a warm bath before bed.

Sleep disordered breathing (apnoea) may impair cognitive ability in older adults. One treatment for this is the continuous positive airway pressure (CPAP) device. This device has the potential to improve cognitive ability at least in the short term, as well as reducing the risk of cardiovascular disease, an important cause of dementia.

What is good-quality sleep?

Good-quality sleep can happen many ways. Humans spend about 30% of their life sleeping. There are a series of cycles that occur during sleep. One sleep cycle takes approximately 90 to 120 minutes and each cycle is comprised of the following four stages (Debanto et al., 2020):

- Stage 1: Light sleep, slowed muscle activity and occasional muscle twitching (1–5 minutes)
- Stage 2: Body enters a more subdued state including a drop in temperature, relaxed muscles, and slowed breathing and heart rate (10–60 minutes).

- Stage 3: Very deep sleep characterized by rhythmic breathing, limited muscle activity, delta waves and cleaning of the brain of toxins (20–40 minutes).
- Stage 4: Rapid Eye Movement (REM) sleep where brainwaves speed up, dreaming occurs, muscles relax, heart rate increases, and breathing becomes rapid and shallow (10–60 minutes).

When people go to sleep, ideally, they proceed uninterrupted through the sleep cycles to get the most out of sleeping. It can take up to six weeks to recover from one night's lost sleep. REM sleep will be longer during each successive stage of sleep if we sleep longer. Waking up earlier interrupts the longest REM stage and can reduce memory and general cognitive ability. Sleep is regulated by certain neurochemicals in the brain which are responsible for controlling different aspects of consciousness and unconsciousness. Changes in sleep occur because of 'homeostasis' ('sleep drive') processes and body clock processes: the technical name for 'body clock' is 'circadian rhythm'. The circadian rhythm is the 24-hour sleep-wake cycle that governs many physiological processes including production of hormones (such as melatonin), gene expression (e.g. information in the gene control production of proteins such as amyloid protein), and body temperature (see Figure 3.3).

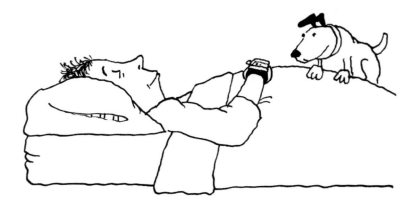

Figure 3.3 Good-quality sleep can happen in many ways.
Source the Optimal Ageing Programme.

Sleep and wake cycles are controlled by the pacemaker activity of the hypothalamus region of the brain. The hypothalamus is the area of the brain concerned with regulating heart rate, body temperature, eating, sleeping, and hormone production. The hormone melatonin assists in being able to go to sleep and stay asleep. Production of this hormone can be disrupted if exposure to light is minimized or non-existent.

When eyes carry light messages to the hypothalamus in the brain, the internal biological clock regulates the circadian rhythm. If the hypothalamus gets mixed messages an unhealthy tug-of-war develops in the body. The mixed messages to the brain occur mostly if the amount of natural light varies too much, for example if people sleep for an hour or two in the middle of the day, and by temperature changes, for example sleeping in a bedroom that is too warm. Mix-ups occur when there is:

- Too much artificial light at night, for example from television, computers, phones, alarm clocks, hallway lights, or streetlights.
- Little or no exposure to light during the day.

The amount of sleep required changes with age. The need to sleep remains the same but the ability to sleep changes. As we live longer, sleep quantity and quality decline, along with the amount of time spent in deep sleep. It takes older adults longer to fall asleep and their sleep is more fragmented, with disturbances occurring more often and earlier. They also tend to awaken less from REM sleep and more from non-REM sleep.

Only 7% of insomnia problems are not related to another existing health problem. The other 93% of reasons for insomnia can include: depression, arthritis, chronic pain, chronic obstructive lung disease, life events, loss of family member, friend or animal, stress, and drugs (beta-blockers, decongestants, antihistamines, cardiac drugs).

Sleep disordered breathing, sometimes called sleep apnoea, increases with age. It is associated with snoring and can cause fragmented or disturbed sleep cycles. Research shows that sleep disordered breathing is often under diagnosed and untreated. The risks for dementia and stroke are increased by sleep disordered breathing. Insomnia, cardiovascular diseases, chronic obstructive pulmonary disease (COPD), sedative drugs, alcohol, smoking, and being overweight increase the risk for sleep disordered breathing.

What is the risk with poor-quality sleep?

Poor-quality or limited sleep is correlated with increased shrinkage atrophy in regions of the brain related to judgement, reasoning, and decision-making. The National Sleep Foundation estimates is that about 40% of the population experience one or more symptoms of insomnia at least three times a week. These are:

- Taking more than 30 minutes to fall asleep.
- Being awake for periods longer than 30 minutes during the night.
- Waking up at least 30 minutes before they had planned.

Also, 20% of the population report being unsatisfied with the quality of their sleep, and 13% report all the symptoms required to diagnose insomnia. Sleep disorders in older adults are not inevitable but are of increased likelihood because older adults typically have two or more long-term conditions and take medication that can disrupt sleep. Insomnia in older adults is associated with falls, poor quality of life, deterioration in balance and ambulation, slower reaction or reflex time, slower wound healing, and an increased risk of dementia.

Sleep disturbance is common in persons living with dementia. About a third of people living with dementia who live in their own homes have sleep problems. People with dementia living in care homes and nursing homes have a higher percentage of sleep problems.

When someone with dementia has sleep problems, different consequences arise. First, there is an increased chance of being admitted to a care home or nursing home. Second, persons with dementia are at higher risk of having their body clock reset for daytime sleep, resulting in night-time wakening and increased 'sundowning', and agitated behaviours at night. Third, people with dementia who have sleep problems also have decreased physical functioning. These problems include balance, falls, fractures, loss of appetite, indigestion, problems with self-care, and lack of strength. People with dementia who have sleep disordered breathing experience poor sleep quality, agitated behaviour at night, and decreased daytime functioning. Finally, persons with dementia and sleep disordered breathing have an impact on the family caregiver's sleep, health, and well-being.

How strong is the evidence that good-quality sleep reduces the risk of dementia?

Sleep studies measure sleep quality either by self-report, actigraphy, or polysomnography. Sleep actigraphs are generally watch-shaped and worn on the wrist of the non-dominant arm. They are useful for determining sleep patterns and circadian rhythms and may be worn for several weeks at a time. Polysomnography is an assessment of how a person sleeps in a sleep clinic overnight. Sleep actigraphs are more affordable than polysomnographs and are particularly advantageous when used in research studies involving large numbers of people.

Polysomnography is a comprehensive recording of the biophysiological changes that occur during sleep. This observation is performed in purpose-built sleep clinics. The 'poly' in polysomnography refers to the multiple measures being taken at the same time while the individual sleeps in the clinic overnight. These measures monitor brain electrical activity (EEG), eye movements (EOG), muscle activity or skeletal muscle activation (EMG), and heart rhythm (ECG).

Studies on how sleep prevents dementia may measure cognitive ability or dementia by self-report of symptoms, and by clinical, neurological, and neuropsychological examinations. In addition, health administrative data is used to identify people with dementia who have received health services for a sleep disorder. Some studies will use two or more of these measures to validate the findings, for example to determine if the different measures classify people the same way regarding their cognitive ability or symptoms of dementia.

Research on populations using sleep self-reports have found a fourfold increase in declining or impaired cognitive ability among people with poor sleep. However, other population research using self-reports have not consistently found this level of an association between sleep and cognitive ability. A good night's sleep is more than just duration. Other important factors include how quickly people fall asleep, the number of times they wake in the night, and whether people are sleeping as deeply as they should be when they cycle through the phases of sleep.

Research shows that sleep is critical for maintaining long-term memories. And sleep is also necessary for removing toxins within the brain.

A recent study of over 10,000 people conducted by Adrian Owen and his colleagues at the Brain and Mind Institute at Western University in Canada, reflects what other population studies have shown. According to a set of 12 well-established tests, cognitive performance was found to be impaired in people who reported typically sleeping less, or more, than seven to eight hours per night, roughly half the sample (Wild et al., 2018).

A recent study of people in the international Alzheimer's Disease Neuroimaging Initiative (ADNI) reported in the journal *Neurology* in 2015 that treating self-reported sleep disordered breathing (apnoea) with a CPAP device delays cognitive difficulties and symptoms of dementia by ten years (Osorio et al., 2015).

Other population studies have shown that people with sleep disordered breathing, involving either cessation of breathing (apnoea), or reduced or shallow breathing (hypo-apnoea) have a greater decline in cognitive ability and an increased risk of dementia. Added to this evidence from population studies, are intervention studies that examine the impact of several methods of improving sleep and reducing the risk of a decline in cognitive ability. Although the trials have been small, computer cognitive training is emerging as a promising intervention for people with insomnia. In other studies, the interventions are exercise, primarily aerobic exercise, bright light therapy, and melatonin therapy.

The CPAP device improves sleep disordered breathing. Trials have shown that in less than three months this device can improve cognitive ability and increase corresponding grey matter volume in hippocampal and frontal regions of the brain. Some trials found cognitive ability changes only, but no reversal of damage to nerves according to assessments using functional MRI imaging technology.

Studies of drugs called acetylcholinesterase inhibitors may improve sleep and cognitive ability. However, these beneficial results must be weighed against the potential side effects of these drugs. In 2020, studies showed evidence that sundowning (agitated behaviour) is reduced with melatonin treatment in persons with dementia. There is uncertainty about the relative size of the benefits and risks associated with common drug treatments including donepezil, fluticasone, benzodiazepine, and non-benzodiazepine hypnotics.

How can risk from lack of sleep be reduced?

Population and intervention studies suggest that insomnia may impair intellectual ability in older adults and treatments such as computer cognitive training have the potential to reduce this effect. The long-term effects, however, of these interventions are unknown. The current evidence-based treatments for sleep disordered breathing are non-drug approaches, such as weight reduction and the use of a CPAP device (see Figure 3.4).

Sleeping pills should not be regarded as the first solution

Sleep medication should only be used as a short-term treatment for insomnia. The dangers of taking sleep medication for prolonged periods of time include possible side effects, addiction to the medication, interactions with other medications, and the fact that sleep medications interfere with all five stages of sleep, particularly REM sleep.

Before deciding to take sleep medication, the following alternative methods could be considered:

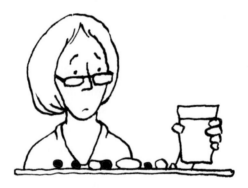

Figure 3.4 Sleep medication should only be used as a short-term treatment of insomnia.
Source the Optimal Ageing Programme.

- Assess the room for sleeping to determine if it is conducive to having a good night's sleep.
- Eliminate computers or televisions in the bedroom. Block additional lighting from streetlights or an alarm clock.
- Reduce noise levels or operate a fan to disguise any background noise. Some people use devices that create sounds of rushing water to help fall asleep. This is called 'white noise'.

Physical activity during the day helps to ensure a good night's sleep. A few hours of daylight exposure are necessary to preserve melatonin to ensure a good night's sleep. Napping during the day should be avoided. Sleep can be improved if the bedroom is cooler (less than 18°C) rather than hotter (more than 20°C).

As sleep is important for better health, like other health improving activities, a routine for sleep should be established. A standard time to go to sleep and a standard time to wake up should be followed. Seven hours of sleep each night should be the goal. Avoid having a light snack, sugar, caffeine, alcohol, nicotine, stimulation from television programmes and computer games, and excessive exercise before going to sleep. However, vigorous exercise is desirable in the morning or late afternoon. Deep breathing before sleep helps to relax and fall asleep.

For families caring for someone living with dementia, pragmatic strategies can be used to help get a better sleep. These strategies include motion activated night lights, a red bulb in night lights, a fan to reduce noises, and having a bath before bed.

A warm bath or holding a warm 'wheat bag' or hot water bottle for half an hour before going to bed can help raise core body temperature. How does it work? Just before falling asleep the body temperature rises for a short period. As the body cools off you feel sleepy. That is why a warm bath before bed can act as an aid in falling asleep.

Am I on the right track with my sleep?

The following checklist can be used to ensure that you are advancing your efforts to have good-quality sleep:

- I am getting seven or more hours of sleep each night and not sleeping more than nine hours.
- I do not wake up during the night more than once.
- I can go to sleep most nights within 30 minutes.
- I do not sleep during the day.

If you can answer yes to all these questions you are doing well if you answer no to one or more than one you need to consider acting.

What sources of support are there for people who want to have good-quality sleep?

In friends and family
The support of friends and family can be helpful in actions to improve your sleep, particularly if they can support the development and implementation of a plan to tackle the causes of poor sleep. Three months of encouragement and support are required for this to be effective.

In the community
'Peers' in the community who also have poor-quality sleep will enable you to relate to and empathize with other people on a level that someone without sleep problems might not be able to do. Talk about sleep problems with friends because they may also be suffering from this common problem.

In the health service
After you have tried to solve your poor-quality sleep, with help from friends and family, and found no community assistance that was helpful it might be time to consult a professional. A physician can identify lifestyle factors or medications that might be getting in the way of better-quality sleep, consider the possibility of sleep apnoea, and refer you for psychological therapy, but most physicians are now wary of prescribing sleeping tablets.

Sleep is very important (see Box 3.2).

Protect your brain from over medication

Modern medicine has had a wonderful impact in the last 50 years, but all healthcare can do harm as well as good and over medication is a preventable cause of dementia.

Polypharmacy refers to the over prescription of drugs. On average, people over the age of 65 are on six drugs a day. Often the physicians who prescribe the drugs do not talk to each other, so the patient gets one drug from the cardiologist, another one from the neurologist, a third from the psychiatrist, and yet another from the endocrinologist. There are 20 drugs that cause memory loss; the leading ones are sleeping pills. Cholesterol lowering medication has also been known to cause memory disturbances on occasion. You need to assess with the assistance of your friends and family and your healthcare practitioners the following:

- Are the drugs you are taking incompatible when taken together?
- Are you able to easily obtain your drugs in your community?
- Are there reasons why you not taking the medication?
- Are you keeping track of how you are doing while you are taking your medications?

How strong is the evidence about the impact of over medication on dementia?

Population surveys have reported that as many as 20% of people reporting memory or confusion can be attributed to the medications they are taking (Lau et al., 2011).

Dementia rarely travels alone. Many people living with dementia also live with one or more other health conditions and the report of the UK All Party Parliamentary group on dementia in 2016 emphasized that:

- 41% have high blood pressure.
- 32% have depression.
- 27% have heart disease.
- 18% have had a stroke or transient ischaemic attack (mini stroke).
- 13% have diabetes.

The implications of this are significant. These are conditions which predominantly affect people as they grow older; we need to ensure that we treat each of these conditions properly, because if we treat blood pressure, for example, the risks of developing dementia decrease. The same can be true for conditions like irregular pulse (atrial fibrillation) and many others. Treating these conditions thus makes sense and the new drugs we use to treat them are both effective and have a lower risk of undesired side effects. But not all drugs are good for you and some can cause problems and not only make dementia worse but make the quality of life for people taking them much worse (see Boxes 3.3 and 3.4).

How could you possibly have too much of something that is good for you? We all remember that as children we were told to eat our vegetables

---

Box 3.4 Free high-quality systematic reviews of the evidence

Anstey, K.J., et al. (2009). Alcohol consumption as a risk factor for dementia and cognitive decline: Meta-analysis of prospective studies. *American Journal of Geriatric Psychiatry*, 17, 542–555.

Blazer, D.G., et al. (2015). Chapter 4B, Risk and protective factors and interventions: Health and medical factors. In: *Cognitive Aging: Progress in Understanding and Opportunities for Action*. Institute of Medicine, National Academies, Washington, DC.

Buckley, J.S. & Salpeter, S.R. (2015). A risk-benefit assessment of dementia medications: Systematic review of the evidence. *Drugs Aging*, 32, 453–467, doi:10.1007/s40266-015-0266-9.

Leelakanok, N., et al. (2019). A systematic review and meta analysis. *Aging Mental Health*, 23(8), 932–941. doi: 10.1080/13607863.2018.1468411. Epub 10 May 2018.

Szekely, C.A., et al. (2004). Nonsteroidal anti-inflammatory drugs for the prevention of Alzheimer's disease: A systematic review. *Neuroepidemiology*, 23, 159–169.

Wang, J., et al. (2015). Anti-inflammatory drugs and risk of Alzheimer's disease: An updated systematic review and meta-analysis. *Journal of Alzheimer's Disease*, 44, 385–396.

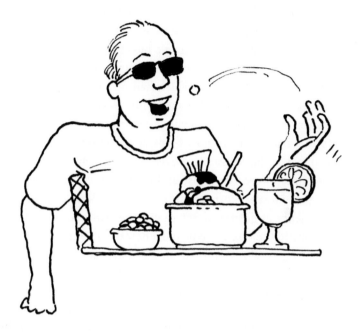

Figure 3.5 *'No matter what I eat doc, isn't there a pill for every disease?'*
Source the Optimal Ageing Programme.

and not to eat too much chocolate and ice cream. No doubt some of us remember thinking as children that life was really unfair and that if chocolate and ice cream were classed as vegetables and carrots and cabbage were desserts, life would be much more fun (see Figure 3.5).

'No matter what I eat doc, isn't there a pill for every disease?'

Medicine has made some extraordinary advances over the years. In the last few centuries life expectancy was much shorter and we really had several limited interventions which we knew really made a difference. The barber surgeon and smooth-talking physicians made a living selling drugs of dubious efficacy, which often caused more unwarranted side effects than beneficial consequences. We used opium to treat pain and distress and sleeplessness and sold it at every street corner. Famous authors like Charles Dickens were addicted to laudanum, a type of opium, as were the poets Elizabeth Browning and John Keats. We have always hoped we would find the 'magic bullet'. Medicine came to the rescue once it became clear that these medicines could cause harm as well as good, and an alternative which had no undesirable addictive side effects was thought to be the answer. In 1864 a German chemist named Baeyer synthesized malonylurea, which in 1903 was then refined into the drugs that we now know as barbiturates (Baeyer gave them this name as they were discovered on St Barbara's day). We believed these drugs were safe to use and addiction was not a problem. It took another 50 years to realize that although these drugs did not cause dependency as quickly as opium did, they still caused addiction. Medicine came to the rescue again and a new drug became the answer to all our problems. This wonder drug was diazepam or Valium. Now we know that this drug has significant adverse effects and needs to be used with caution. We certainly were not aware of that then. Thus, the cycle repeats itself again and again and perhaps it is better if we start to think differently about how we use drugs most effectively and the context in which we use them.

We have always hoped that a magic little pill will cure all our ills. It would allow us to lie on the sofa all day, eating all the chocolate and ice cream we wanted whilst drinking wine and smoking cigars. Taking the miracle pill every day to stop or reverse disease would allow us to continue to do whatever we wished, negating the effects of a whole lifetime of indulgence. Sadly, this is not the case. What we do today influences tomorrow. What we did yesterday and even choices made during childhood have an effect. We need to invest in our health and wellness through the whole of our lives, not wait for something to go wrong then try to do everything to turn the clock back. The good news is, it is never too late to start, and it is better to start today than wait until tomorrow.

So why should we be wary of over medication and what does this have to do with dementia?

An example that really illustrates questionable prescribing of drugs is the use of 'atypical antipsychotics' for people living with dementia. These are a group of drugs which are major tranquillizers and used in the treatment of psychiatric illnesses. They were used extensively in care homes and nursing homes to manage agitation in people living with dementia and inevitably ended up being used like 'chemical coshes' in some instances as they made people much more docile as well as sleepy. Although they of course still have a use in people with psychiatric illnesses, including people with dementia, their use now is more selective and invariably they tend to be used by specialists in selected cases. Previously they were used indiscriminately as their calming effect on people who took them made them much easier to manage. Sadly, in many instances, they also made their lives much more miserable. Though people may have looked calmer and more vacant, their feelings of agitation could well have persisted, they just could not show it. The indiscriminate use of these drugs was discontinued over a period of a few weeks and everyone was worried that there would be hell to pay once people who had been heavily sedated 'woke up'. Nothing could be further from the truth. There were numerous examples of people who communicated again with relatives and carers after months or years of being uncommunicative and not even recognizing their husbands or wives. Thus, we need to be careful not to overmedicate ourselves, but know which drugs can cause problems.

What needs to be remembered is that all drugs need to be used with caution as we live longer. Our livers and kidneys that are the engines that help us excrete and detoxify the drugs we take are inevitably not quite as efficient as they were when we were 20 years younger. If we are living with mild cognitive impairment (MCI), the side effects of drugs can also be magnified and in some cases it has been reported that people were labelled as living with dementia when actually they were 'overdosing' on some drugs either because they were on the wrong dose or because the side effects for them were particularly severe.

Any medications that have a psychoactive or hypnotic effect, such as tranquillizers and strong pain killers, should be used with caution in people living with dementia. Some, such as benzodiazepines and barbiturates, and antipsychotics, can cause drowsiness, confusion, increased cognitive impairment, slowed reaction, and worsening balance, leading to falls. Sleeping pills usually have the same effects. Other drugs that we do not think of as influencing cognitive function can also be potentially harmful. Simple antihistamines that many take for hay fever, for example, can cause drowsiness and confusion and are best avoided. There are better alternatives now, such as less-sedating antihistamines. These class of drugs are also used for nausea as antiemetics (to stop feelings of sickness and wanting to vomit). There are alternatives that can be used which do not predispose to confusion and drowsiness. One over-the-counter antihistamine medication that is commonly used by older adults in the community setting and that worsens cognition is diphenhydramine.

There are other classes of drugs we need to use with caution and, if possible, avoid in favour of alternatives. For example, disopyramide is a drug used to treat some types of atrial fibrillation (irregular heartbeat) and can exacerbate dementia, as can drugs we use as antispasmodics for people suffering from irritable bowel syndrome and drugs to treat parkinsonism. Drugs used to treat symptoms of an enlarged prostate and urinary incontinence can also have a similar effect.

Antispasmodics are a group of drugs used to treat irritable bowel syndrome. This is a very common condition affecting many people and often presenting with symptoms like wind, bloating, and changes to bowel habit. There are many drugs used to treat this condition which have anticholinergic effects, namely which limit the effect and duration of action of the neurotransmitter acetylcholine. Acetylcholine is a neurotransmitter, a transmitter of impulses between nerves. We know that impairment of acetylcholine transmission plays a key role in the development of dementia. In fact, many of the drugs commonly used to treat dementia like donepezil, rivastigmine, and galantamine are cholinesterase inhibitors because cholinesterase destroys acetylcholine and therefore reduces transmission. This means that the drugs we commonly use to treat dementia increase the level and duration of action of the neurotransmitter acetylcholine, thus improving the connectivity within the brain.

Caution also needs to be exercised when treating parkinsonism. This is a condition which can be associated with certain types of dementia, which means that treatment should be planned by specialists. Drugs commonly used like benztropine, procyclidine, and trihexyphenidyl all have anticholinergic effects. We now tend to use these drugs only in selected cases, for example in tremor, in early disease, and in people with good cognitive function. In other cases, levodopa is often used.

Urinary incontinence is a common condition in older age groups and here also the treatment that is often used relies on the anticholinergic effect of the drugs as this helps the incontinence and improves the muscle tone in the bladder. There are some alternative drugs that can be used, but drugs like oxybutynin and flavoxate are also known to have marked anti-cholinergic effects.

Prostatism (or symptoms associated with an enlarged prostate) is a particularly common symptom in men growing older. These manifests itself as wanting to urinate frequently, often waking at night to do so, as well as urgency, diminished urinary stream, and other symptoms. Here treatment is also often affected, using drugs like tolterodine that is an anticholinergic.

Excessive alcohol substantially increases the risk of dementia, as found in a 2018 study in France examining frequency of alcohol use disorders among 1,109,343 people with dementia discharged from hospital. The authors conclude that heavy drinking is detrimentally related to dementia risk, whatever the dementia type for four reasons. First, ethanol and its metabolite acetaldehyde have a direct neurotoxic effect, leading to permanent structural and functional brain damage. Second, heavy drinking is associated with thiamine deficiency, leading to Wernicke–Korsakoff syndrome. Third, heavy drinking is a risk factor for other conditions that can also damage the brain, such as epilepsy, head injury, and hepatic encephalopathy in patients with cirrhotic liver disease. Fourth, heavy drinking is indirectly associated with vascular dementia because of the associations of heavy drinking with vascular risk factors such as high blood pressure, haemorrhagic stroke, atrial fibrillation, and heart failure.

The message is a simple one: despite the complexities of the science, any drug that can make you feel drowsy and is psychoactive and works on the brain needs to be taken with caution. Even drugs which can cause drowsiness but are taken for other reasons like antihistamines for hay fever or muscle relaxants to stop spasmodic conditions need to be monitored carefully or avoided if possible.

There are some other drugs that can mimic the development of dementia as well as making symptoms worse in people living with it. These are drugs that are used for common conditions but drugs that have a narrow therapeutic window. In other words drugs that do you good if you take them at the right dose for your body, weight, and age but do you harm if you take too much of them or lack the good liver and kidney function to excrete them. A good example here is thyroxin.

Thyroxin is a drug that is used effectively in treating low thyroid function and it works well when you take the right dose. If you take the wrong dose it causes harm, both if you take too little, when you are prone to develop myxoedema, or too much, when you will develop symptoms of thyrotoxicosis. In both these instances cognitive effects can lead to symptoms that can mimic those of dementia. Similarly, drugs like vitamin D, which are used for calcium absorption and metabolism need to be monitored carefully, as disordered calcium metabolism can also mimic dementia.

Am I on the right track with my pill taking?

There is a way to be safe and this is to take medication only when you are advised to or need to, ensure you take the right dose and avoid doing yourself harm through overdose. Just follow these steps for safer drug use:

- Medication is not a panacea, but part, sometimes an important part, of what someone needs to do to reduce the risk of disease or reduce the impact of disease. If you have high blood pressure and are overweight, it is very important to take your prescribed medication, but also to manage your weight, to avoid adding salt to your food, and to exercise.
- Medication needs to be monitored. Your doctor will help you here. Too much medicine can be directly harmful and too little will treat the underlying condition ineffectively. Your doctor will advise you to get regular checks. It is in your interest to get these done, despite the extra effort in doing this.
- Ageing can affect the ability to manage medication as we live longer, because some of our bodily functions and organs also change our tolerance to drugs, for example changes in the liver and kidneys. Thus, just because you are on the right dose in January does not mean the dose is right in June.
- Watch out if an acute illness occurs. Illness, even common illnesses, can change our tolerance. Simple urinary tract infections in older people often cause confusion and inevitably exacerbate any side

effects. The same is true in conditions like heart failure, a condition where the heart does not act as an efficient pump.

- Medication needs to be taken as it is prescribed. It is really tempting not to take a drug if you are feeling fine, but you are prescribed it for a reason, omitting doses can be a problem and lead to under treatment.

- Remember not all over-the-counter medications are safe for you to take. Even simple antihistamines can cause problems. If in doubt always ask the pharmacist, they are experts on drugs and their side effects.

- Think long term. Some medication may give you the illusion of short-term gain but will give you long-term pain. Sleeping tablets are a notable example. They may give you the illusion of sleep, although you will not experience the restorative effects of deep sleep. They cause chemical unconsciousness in the short term and lead inevitably to habituation. The last thing you need is to be addicted and not be able to sleep, which is the inevitable story of many a person who started taking these medicines for convenience.

- Do not get over obsessional about taking medication. Everything in life is about managing risk. Not crossing a road is less risky than crossing it, but this does not mean we never cross a road. There is a balance of risk and reward in everything, including medication. Speak to your doctor or pharmacist about this and research medicines online. There are some good websites that are factual and written in plain English, especially NHS Choices or Medline Plus, produced by the National Library for Health in Washington, DC.

- Just because something is not a marketed as a drug does not mean it does not have the effects of drugs. Alcohol is bought at the supermarket, but we all know that having too much can cause problems in the short, medium, and long term.

- Be wary of 'food supplements' and unlicensed products you can find advertised in glossy magazines that promise all sorts of good things if you take them. Some can be positively harmful; others can interact with medicines you take, and all of them potentially cost you money. You can do yourself a favour by saving the money and going on holiday—the effect of that will probably be better for you and be more sustained.

What sources of support are there for people who want to avoid over medication?

In friends and family
Friends and family can be helpful if you have concerns about taking medications and you should be encouraged to have a conversation about your medicines. By understanding your existing routine for managing your medicines, it may be possible to identify potential problems and how to overcome these. They can also help with opening the packages some drugs are in, reading small print on drug labels, and reminding you take your medication.

In the community
Rather than seeking out another pill to cure your next ailment, look around in your community for other approaches to improving your health and quality of life. Pain control is a good example of where alternative non-pharmacological approaches are important and eliminate the risk of becoming addicted to one of the pain management drugs that are dispensed by healthcare professionals. For example, pain can be controlled with relaxation techniques to help you relieve stress and decrease pain. These techniques include:

- Aromatherapy.
- Deep breathing, testing your muscles, and then relaxing.
- Medication and yoga to help your mind and body relax.
- Guided imagery teaches you to imagine a picture in your mind. You learn to focus on the picture instead of your pain. It may help you learn how to change the way your body senses and responds to pain.
- Music may help increase energy levels and improve your mood. It may help reduce pain by triggering your body to release endorphins. These are natural chemicals, produced by the body that decrease pain.
- Biofeedback helps your body respond differently to the stress of being in pain.

- Self-hypnosis is a way to direct your attention to something other than your pain. Acupuncture therapy uses thin needles to balance energy channels in the body and this may help reduce pain and other symptoms.

In the health service

One important principle is that the people most at risk may be the group that is least able to ask for a review of their medication. Physicians now have a clear responsibility to review the medication of people getting multiple prescribed drugs, with many people on five, ten, or even more prescriptions. The process is called de-prescribing and if you are on a number of different drugs that have been pre-scribed by different specialists, or are helping or supporting someone who is, you should ask the general practitioner for a review of all the medication.

Everyone should check with their doctor before mixing medicines, in-cluding over-the-counter medications. In addition to medications that physicians prescribe to patients, over-the-counter drugs can also cause problems. For example, your doctor can review your heart medications and avoid prescribing heart medications that when mixed with aspirin and supplements such as omega-3 fish oil and garlic are known to cause problems with cognitive functioning. Healthcare practitioners are in-structed through guidelines to consider the following issues in a hand-book from the US Agency for Healthcare Research and Quality called *Patient Safety and Quality*, by Ronda Hughes:

- Whether the drugs you are taking are incompatible (medication reconciliation).
- How and where you obtain your drugs (medical procurement).
- Whether or not you are taking the medication and the reasons why (intentional non-adherence).
- Keeping track of how you are doing while taking your medications (ongoing monitoring).

Medicines are part of the reason that modern healthcare has had a tre-mendous impact on death and disability, but remember all healthcare can do harm as well as good.

Get more active and physically fitter

Maintaining and indeed increasing your levels of physical activity is an effective way of reducing the risk of dementia. Increasing physical activity has both direct and indirect benefits on the brain. Brain tissue responds directly to physical activity. The indirect effect is by making keeping the oxygen rich blood supply flowing freely. There is strong evidence that increasing activity slows decline in brain function.

How strong is the evidence about the risk from inactivity?

As with all factors related to the environment we live in and how we adapt to it the evidence relates to two questions:

- How strong is the evidence that physical inactivity is associated with an increased risk of dementia?
- How strong is the evidence that increasing the amount of activity you take will reduce your risk of dementia?

Before addressing the first question it is helpful to consider how physical activity could affect the risk of dementia, because an understanding of the possible ways in which inactivity increases risk has influenced the design of the different types of research that have been undertaken. Perhaps the most obvious means of risk reduction is by maintaining a good blood supply to the brain. Vascular dementia is the medical term used to define dementia in which the loss of brain tissue is the result of damage to the arteries supplying the brain, for example the arteries in the neck (discussed in the next chapter).

Physical activity keeps arteries healthy both directly and indirectly. The direct effect is only now being understood, but it does appear that physical activity can prevent inflammation in the arteries, which leads to atherosclerosis and the furring up of the arteries with atheroma, a porridge-like substance made up of fat and inflammatory tissue. The fatty changes all have the same cause, intake of excessive calories from food and under expenditure of calories through activity.

These conditions, hypercholesterolaemia and pre-diabetes, for example, have names that sound as though they are real diseases like rheumatoid arthritis or tuberculosis. However, they are just the consequence of our modern environment dominated by cars, the Internet, the computer screen, the desk job, and an environment in which high calorie food is universally available and cheap. No one would want to return to the days in which back-breaking work was the norm for the poorer people in society. Even the man digging up the road performs less physical activity than previously, through sitting on his bottom and using his thumbs to control a mechanical digger. The sedentary lifestyle is now almost universal, but it does influence blood pressure, blood sugar, and blood lipids.

Everyone has cholesterol, lipids, and sugar in their bloodstream, and everyone has a blood pressure. They are all essential for life. However, when inactivity, often aggravated by consuming more calories than are needed, increases the levels of these chemicals then they change from being essential for life to becoming a risk to health and life. They are risk factors not diseases, but the medical profession has given them names as though they were diseases like tuberculosis, such as:

- Hypercholesterolaemia.
- Type 2 diabetes.
- High blood pressure.

These increase the risk of vascular dementia, but evidence that physical activity can reduce the risk of or prevent atherosclerosis by modifying these factors is strong. Most of the studies so far have looked at the impact on heart disease, but increasingly there is evidence of an impact on dementia also. Even more exciting, perhaps, is the more recent research on the direct impact of exercise on the brain. In 2015, Harvard Medical School, one of the world's top medical schools, published a Special Health Report on *Walking for Health* and included a fascinating section on the benefits of walking on the brain, an excerpt of which has been included below:

'Walking helps maintain brain volume and reduces memory problems in people who have mild cognitive impairment or Alzheimer's disease, according to a ten-year study from the University of Pittsburgh (a decline in brain volume means that brain cells are dying). Even healthy adults benefited if they walked six miles a week. In particular, the hippocampus—a section of the brain that's crucial to memory— normally shrinks by 1% to 2% a year in older adults without cognitive impairment. In a study related to the one above, researchers found that walking six miles a week for a year not only offset the shrinkage, it actually increased hippocampal volume by 2%. Walking also appears to enhance brain connectivity, so a person is better at planning, prioritizing, strategizing, and multitasking. When 65 sedentary people, ages 59 to 80, walked for 40 minutes three times a week for a year, brain scans showed greater connectivity, according to a University of Illinois study.'

(Harvard Health Publishing, 2018)

This means that walking can prevent not only the diseases with which exercise is usually associated, heart disease for example, it can also help reduce the risk of the condition that people wish to avoid more than any other—dementia, not only by improving the blood flow to the brain but also by a direct effect on both the grey and the white tissues.

The Academy of Medical Royal Colleges report on *Exercise—the Miracle Cure* concluded that: 'the evidence is fairly consistent in quoting reduced risks of dementia at 20–50%' (from physical activity). This has been reported before and the usually cautious, and prestigious *Journal of the American Medical Association* published evidence in 2004 that walking can prevent loss of intellectual or cognitive ability. The research reports stated that: 'Findings suggest that walking is associated with a reduced risk of dementia. Promoting active lifestyles in physically capable men could help later life cognitive function' (Abbott et al., 2004). This journal also reported that: 'Long term physical activity including walking, is associated with significantly better cognitive function and less cognitive decline in older women' (Weuve et al., 2004).

How can you reduce your risk from inactivity?

The evidence that increasing exercise reduces risk is now compelling the National Institute of Health and Care Excellence (NICE), which reviews evidence on all topics for the NHS. NICE expressed the results of their review very closely by saying that people in midlife could 'delay or prevent the onset' of dementia. The evidence comes from reviews of randomized controlled trials, some of which study exercise on its own or focus on exercise combined with other interventions which reduce the risk of vascular disease, for example the Finnish Geometric Intervention Study to Prevent Cognitive Impairment and Disability trial (referred to as the FINGER trial). This type of trial is only feasible in well-organized countries like Finland. Their conclusion published in the *Lancet* in 2018 was that: 'Improvement … was 25% to 150% better in the intervention than in the control group' (Rosenberg et al., 2018).

The authors also point out that these effects might be 'conservative', namely an underestimate of the true size of the benefit because of the way the study was designed.

The Harvard Medical School *Guide to Coping with Alzheimer's Disease* also describes the benefits of exercise for people who carry the E4 allele of the APOE gene which increases the risk of Alzheimer's disease. In one study, people who carried this gene had brain scans carried out over an 18-month period. The research subjects who did not have an exercise programme showed a 3% decline in brain tissue in a part of the brain called the hippocampus. Those who engaged in a regular exercise programme showed no such decline. The message is clear: we need to exercise more, not only because of the effect of this on individuals, but also because it gets us out of our shells and enables us to socialize. More and more organizations are instituting walking clubs and exercise clubs. Not only does participating in these activities cut our risk of developing dementia by increasing activity, but it also gives us an opportunity to interact with others and decrease levels of social isolation, tackling another risk factor for dementia. A true win/win (see Box 3.5).

Watch this space; developments that do not yet have evidence of effectiveness

The preoccupation with the study of amyloid, tau protein, and fibrillary tangles, has consumed the time of researchers and the resources of both charities and pharmaceutical companies committed to finding a cure for Alzheimer's disease. This research is now coming to an end. Enthusiasm

---

Box 3.5   Free high-quality systematic reviews of the evidence

---

Beckett, M.W., Ardern, C.I., & Rotondi, M.A. (2015). A meta-analysis of prospective studies on the role of physical activity and the prevention of Alzheimer's disease in older adults. *BMC Geriatrics*, 15, 9.

Blondell, S.J., Hammersley-Mather, R., & Veerman, J.L. (2014). Does physical activity prevent cognitive decline and dementia? A systematic review and meta-analysis of longitudinal studies. *BMC Public Health*, 14, 510.

Deckers, K., van Boxtel, M.P.J., Schiepers, O.J.G., de Vugt, M., et al. (2015). Target risk factors for dementia prevention: A systematic review and Delphi consensus study of the evidence from observational studies. *International Journal of Geriatric Psychiatry*, 30, 234–246.

Global Council on Brain Health (2016). The brain-body connection: GCBH recommendations on physical activity and brain health. Available at: www.GlobalCouncilOnBrainHealth.org

Hamer, M. & Chida, Y. (2009). Physical activity and risk of neurodegenerative disease: A systematic review of prospective evidence. *Psychological Medicine*, 39, 3–11.

Santos-Lozano, A., Pareja-Galeano, H., Sanchis-Gomar, F., Quinddos-Rubial, M., Fiuza-Luces, C., Cristi-Montero, C., et al. (2016). Physical activity and Alzheimer disease: A protective association. *Mayo Clinic Proceedings*, 91, 999–1020.

Xu, W., Wang, H.F., Wan, Y., Tan, C.C., Yu, J.T., & Tan, L. (2017). Leisure time physical activity and dementia risk: A dose-response meta-analysis of prospective studies. *BMJ Open*, 7, e014706.

---

has waned recently, not because the money has run out but because it has become apparent that the task is much more complex than the search for a single cure for a single disease.

One of the benefits of the investment in a better understanding of the genetics of Alzheimer's disease has been the belated realization of the fact that a disease entity has been described by a single clinician and reinforced by no more than human perception of changes seen through a microscope. This is how Dr Alzheimer discovered or, perhaps more accurately, invented the disease, probably better considered to be a group of related conditions. Each of the 'conditions formerly considered as the single entity called Alzheimer's disease', which is a more long-winded but accurate term, may have different causes and therefore require a different prevention and treatment strategy. In addition to the growing interest in inflammation described in the previous chapter, three other themes are emerging from research as potential risk factors and therefore as potential opportunities for further reducing the risk by protecting the brain tissue. These factors are pollution, diet, and gum disease.

Pollution

The effects of pollution on health are difficult to assess except where there is a direct effect, for example the effect of smog on the lungs. There are multiple chemicals and particulates involved, often in small concentrations, and they are often combined with other risk factors. For example, pollution is often higher in areas in which people with high levels of deprivation live. New technology allows the detection of new types of particles in small concentrations as one paper published in the journal *Proceedings of the National Academy of Sciences* described: 'Our results indicate that magnetite nanoparticles in the atmosphere can enter the human brain, where they might pose a risk to human health, including conditions such as Alzheimer's disease.' Concern about pollution in general will see this subject studied more and the effect on the brain will be one aspect of this research (Peters et al., 2019).

Pesticides

Evidence suggests that lifelong cumulative exposure to pesticides may generate lasting toxic effects on the central nervous system and contribute to developing dementia (Yan et al., 2016).

Anti-ageing diets

From time to time some food stuff receives publicity as 'the means of preventing dementia' but it is more important to watch the research on diets that appear to reduce the impact of the whole ageing process. In the next chapter we will praise the contribution that the Mediterranean diet can make to reducing disease of blood vessels, protecting the blood supply to the brain. But recent research suggests that the Mediterranean diet is not an anti-ageing diet in the way that the diets of people livening in Okinawa and, perhaps surprisingly, Scandinavia are. The Japanese diet is of course excellent, but the island of Okinawa's diet includes the nutrient-rich purple sweet potato, often eaten in place of rice and Okinawans tend to eat less fish, meat, rice, and sugar (and fewer calories overall) than those in other parts of Japan.

People are now studying the Scandinavian diet and found they cook with canola oil, also called rapeseed oil, which contains more omega-3 fatty acids than olive oil. As well as eating more seafood, and relatively less meat and dairy, they also eat certain fruits called lingonberries, lots of potatoes, nuts, and wholegrain bread, including rye bread.

There is a move now to relate these findings to a new approach which goes further than the Mediterranean diet and is called the Mediterranean-DASH-diet Intervention for Neurodegenerative Delay diet (or MIND diet). Scientists developed it by combining features from those healthy dietary patterns in the Mediterranean diet and the Dietary Approaches to Stop Hypertension diet (or DASH diet) and incorporating specific dietary strategies shown to support brain health. For example, it calls for at least six servings a week of leafy green vegetables and at least two servings a week of strawberries or blueberries (Lehert et al., 2015; Van de Rest et al., 2015). These diets can reduce the risk of type 2 diabetes and the risk of inflammation. Another topic to watch as it moves from being of interest to academic biologists studying how our bodies, designed for stone age survival cope with the post stone age in which food is more than plentiful, activity less than necessary, and stress often occurs in situations in which you just have to sit and take it, and as a consequence, develop inflammation.

Large companies have developed marketing for specific dietary supplements and vitamins, but there is no strong evidence to support their use, and therefore their purchase (better to spend money on a trainer).

A report from the Global Council on Brain Health, sponsored by the excellent American Association of Retired Persons (AARP) in 2019 was clear on this issue. However, this remains an important area of research with some encouraging results. For example, the Oxford Project To investigate Memory and Ageing (OPTIMA) carried out an intervention trial (VITACOG) in 2004–2009 in Oxford for people with MCI. During the trial half the subjects were given a mixture of vitamin B (folic acid and vitamins B6 and B12) for two years. A reduction in the rate of atrophy was found in the B vitamin group that was greatest in those with high plasma homocysteine at baseline. The vitamin B treatment also slowed cognitive decline (AARP website).

Gum disease

After the age of about 60, people who want to keep a lovely smile need to shift their focus from their teeth to their gums. No matter how well the teeth are kept, they will simply drop out unless the gums are kept in good health. The main cause of this is periodontal infection, or gum infection to use an everyday term. The first problem that develops is plaque and bacteria feed on the plaque and then invade the tissues below, weakening the roots of the teeth, which may simply drop out or must be removed. However, what is also emerging is the fact that one of the species of bacteria called *Porphyromonas gingivalis*, is now being found in the brain, particularly in those parts of the brain in which Alzheimer's disease occurs first. The hippocampus is one of these locations and is associated with the changes in amyloid and tau proteins which were regarded as the cause of Alzheimer's disease.

The respected journal *Scientific American* reviewed this topic in January 2019, describing how: 'Multiple teams have been researching *Porphyromonas gingivalis*, the main bacterium involved in gum disease, which is a known risk factor for Alzheimer's. So far, teams have found that *P. gingivalis* invades and inflames brain regions affected by Alzheimer's; that gum infections can worsen symptoms in mice genetically engineered to have Alzheimer's; and that it can cause Alzheimer-like brain inflammation, neural damage, and amyloid plaques in healthy mice' (*New Scientist*, website).

This is a topic of great interest to researchers (Harding et al., 2017; Kramer et al., 2014; Singhrao et al., 2015; Tzenget al., 2016). No one is yet claiming that by preventing or treating gum disease dementia can be prevented. However, because there is such a strong desire to keep one's teeth, there are several motivations to adopt these measures anyway. These include adopting the benefits of high technology, such as the electronic toothbrush, as well as appointments with dental hygienists, who make people are aware of gum disease as a problem and encourage them want to tackle it by brushing their gums, as well as teeth, for at least four minutes a day. Debora Mackenzie, the author of the *New Science* article gave it the title: 'We may finally know the cause of Alzheimer's disease and how to stop it.' We know about its link in mice through testing, but the link in humans has yet to be proven and researchers are looking hard at this possible risk factor.

The search for drugs to treat or prevent Alzheimer's disease will continue

There have been many disappointments in the search for drugs to treat or prevent Alzheimer's disease, but this must continue. The focus is usually on two types of damage that can be seen in the brains of people with Alzheimer's disease. These are referred to as neurofibrillary tangles in a protein called hyperphosphorylated tau and solid plaques of a protein called beta amyloid. Vaccines have been developed but have only been tested on mice so far.

There will be reports of 'breakthroughs' and developments in the press, but our judgement is that vitally important though such research will be for the next five years, the knowledge summarized in this book about the prevention of the causes of dementia other than Alzheimer's disease will be the basis of both individual and social action.

References

Abbott, R.D., et al. (2004). Walking and dementia in physically capable men. *Journal of American Medical Association*, 12, 1447–1453.

American Association of Retired Persons (2020). *Global Council on Brain Health. Nutrition and Brain Health.* Available at: https://www.aarp.org/health/brain-health/global-council-on-brain-health/nutrition/

Becker, E., et al. (2018). Anxiety as a risk factor of Alzheimer's disease and vascular dementia. *British Journal of Psychiatry*, 5, 654–660.

Debanto J, Suni E. How sleep works. Sleep Foundation. Seattle. October 20, 2020. (https://www.sleepfoundation.org/how-sleep-works/stages-of-sleep).

Harding, A., et al. (2017). Can better management of periodontal disease delay the onset and progression of Alzheimer's disease? *Journal of Alzheimer's Disease*, 2, 337–348.

Harvard Health Publishing (2018). *Walking for Health*. Harvard Health Publishing, Cambridge, MA.

Kramer, A.R., et al. (2014). Periodontal disease associates with higher brain amyloid load in normal elderly. *Neurobiology of Aging*, 2, 627–633.

Lau, D.T., Mercaldo, N.D., Harris, A.T., Trffschuh, E., et al. (2011). Polypharmacy and potentially inappropriate medication use among community-dwelling elders with dementia. *Alzheimer Disease Association Disorders*, 1, 56–63.

Lehert, P., et al. (2015). Individually modifiable risk factors to ameliorate cognitive aging: A systematic review and meta-analysis. *Climacteric*, 5, 678–689.

Mackenzie, D. (2019). We may finally know the cause of Alzheimer's disease and how to stop it. *New Scientist*. Available at: https://www.newscientist.com/article/2191814-we-may-finally-know-what-causes-alzheimers-and-how-to-stop-it/

Osorio, R.S., Gumb, T., Pirraglia, E., Varga, A.W., et al. (2015). Sleep-disordered breathing advances cognitive decline in the elderly. *Neurology*, 19, 1964–1971.

Peters, R., et al. (2019). Air pollution and dementia: A systematic review. *Journal of Alzheimer's Disease*, S1, S145–S163.

Rosenberg, A., Ngandu, T., Rusanen, M., Antikainen, R., et al. (2018). Multidomain lifestyle intervention benefits a large elderly population at risk for cognitive decline and dementia regardless of baseline characteristics: The FINGER trial. *Alzheimer's Dementia*, 3, 263–270.

Singhrao, S.K., et al. (2015). *Porphyromonas gingivalis* periodontal infection and its putative links with Alzheimer's disease. *Hindawi*, |Article ID 137357.

Tzeng, N.-S., et al. (2016). Are chronic periodontitis and gingivitis associated with dementia? A nationwide, retrospective, matched-cohort study in Taiwan. *Neuroepidemiology*, 2, 82–93.

Van de Rest, O., et al. (2015). Dietary patterns, cognitive decline, and dementia: A systematic review. *Advances in Nutrition*, 2, 154–168.

Weuve, J., et al. (2004). Physical activity, including walking, and cognitive function in older women. *Journal of American Medical Association*, 12, 1454.

Wild, C.J., et al. (2018). Dissociable effects of self-reported daily sleep duration on high-level cognitive abilities. *Sleep*, 41(12), zsy182.

Yan, D., et al. (2016). Pesticide exposure and risk of Alzheimer's disease: A systematic review and meta-analysis. *Scientific Reports*, 6(32222).

4

Maintain and Increase Blood Supply to the Brain

Everything that is written and said about the prevention of heart disease or the prevention of stroke appears to be equally relevant to the prevention of dementia. These are presented as the following key points:

- Increase physical activity (covered in the previous chapter).
- Rebalance your diet.
- Keep your sugar low, avoid type 2 diabetes.
- Keep your cholesterol low.
- Stop smoking.
- Keep your blood pressure low.
- Keep your weight down.
- Find out if you have atrial fibrillation and get it treated.
- Check if you have had a transient ischaemic attack (TIA for short) the word 'ischaemic' being Greek for 'without blood'.

Vascular dementia is caused by damage to the arteries of the brain and this damage is caused by the same risk factors that cause heart disease, because what is called heart disease is in fact disease of all the arteries, including the arteries of the brain. Therefore, the steps taken to reduce the risk of heart disease also reduce the risk of dementia. In addition, most of the people who have one of the different types of dementia, including those with a specific name such as Alzheimer's disease, also have some disease in their arteries. This is because almost everyone in a modern, industrialized society has some degree of arterial disease; atherosclerosis is the name of the underlying disease process.

You don't often see brain in butchers' windows in our communities, or indeed on the menu, but that is a simple cultural quirk (see Figure 4.1).

Increase your Brainability—and Reduce your Risk of Dementia. Charles Alessi, Larry W. Chambers, and Muir Gray, Oxford University Press. © Oxford University Press 2021. DOI: 10.1093/oso/9780198860341.003.0004

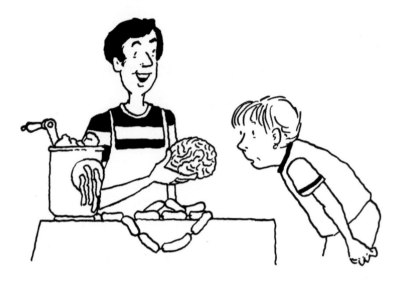

Figure 4.1 Brains look like a lunar landscape with coils and deep gulches between them with mostly grey matter on the surface.
Source the Optimal Ageing Programme.

Cervello is popular in Italy and many other countries. If you can find a brain to look at, do so, or ask the butcher (who may be putting it into the occasional sausage if he feels his customers are too sensitive to see the organ itself) to show you a brain. These would, of course, be from a cow.

Take the opportunity to study an animal brain in your local butcher's shop

The surface of the brain is like a lunar landscape with coils and deep gulches between them. When the brain is cut across there is a familiar pattern in all species. The brain tissue itself is mostly white, with about a centimetre of grey matter on the surface—the grey matter, the little grey cells of Hercule Poirot. It was thought at one time that the grey matter was the clever part of the brain, but we now know that both grey and white are of vital importance. Arteries are ubiquitous in the brain and divide again and again into smaller and smaller branches.

In butchers' windows the brain is strikingly different from the liver, kidney, or muscle, such as that in the fillet steak. Theses tissues are red and obviously blood filled, but the brain, with its vast array of arteries, depends on its blood supply at least as much as those other organs. You can manage fine with just one kidney or if one third of your liver must be removed because a cancer secondary has landed up there. However, every part of the brain is of importance, and if any part of its oxygen-rich, arterial blood supply is interrupted, serious problems occur, depending on which part of the brain is affected.

If a major artery is blocked or if the artery bursts the result is called a stroke and is usually made obvious by paralysis of one side of the body. Sometimes the blockage is small, temporary, and disappears after the patient experiences weakness, numbness or paralysis in the face, arm, or leg, slurred or garbled speech or difficulty understanding others, or blindness in one or both eyes, or double vision. This is called a transient ischaemic attack (TIA) or mini stroke. If the TIA happens in a part of the brain that controls other functions, some aspect of memory for example, then the event may pass without notice but if lots of little blockages occur the consequences are serious, vascular dementia.

Doctors have long suspected the fact that some people developed dementia because they had experienced lots of infarcts. Infarcts being small areas of dead tissue, killed by lack of blood supply. Each of these infarcts would have affected parts of the brain that did not control muscle movement and therefore did not cause any signs of weakness. They were too small to be seen until, that is, the development of magnetic resonance imaging (MRI), which is much more powerful than traditional X-rays. These allowed research radiologists, such as the team at the University of Edinburgh, led by Professor Joanna Wardlow, to demonstrate the presence of tiny flecks of white in the brains of people with dementia. This demonstrated that vascular dementia was a real entity. These tiny areas of damage were found everywhere in the brain. This demonstrated that vascular dementia was a real entity and is recognized as a contributor to small strokes and silent strokes.

The circulation system is like a central heating system. In a central heating system there is a boiler with pump; the heart is the pump in the circulation system. The pump in a central heating system circulates energy, produced by burning coal, oil, or gas in a boiler. In the body, the energy is produced from carbohydrates burned in all the tissues, with oxygen drawn in from the lungs and carried by the blood to the tissues through the arteries. Unlike the central heating system, the energy is not generated in the central boiler but in the tissues of the body, by the interaction between oxygen and carbohydrate. This happens everywhere, for example in the muscles. In the brain, any interruption in the flow of oxygen results in an interruption in the production of energy, and tissues which are starved of energy die.

There are three ways in which the circulation of blood to the brain tissue can be cut off. An artery may:

- Become progressively furred up, just like a water pipe, by the development of a substance often described by pathologists as 'porridgy' in the walls of the artery. This process of narrowing the arteries is called atherosclerosis and is the result of several factors, one of which is inflammation.
- Simply burst, usually due to a combination of high blood pressure, and the weakening of the artery wall that results from atherosclerosis.
- Become blocked by a clot of blood that has developed in the heart and is then carried through arteries. These arteries become smaller and smaller until they are too small for the clot to pass through, causing it to stick there. This blocks the supply of oxygen to the part of the brain that depends on that artery for its oxygen supply. The reason a clot forms is usually if there is an irregular rhythm of the heart, a disorder called atrial fibrillation. If the clot is a big one, it will stick sooner, as arteries divide again and again into smaller and smaller branches. The result is a stroke, which may be fatal or paralyse half the body. If the clot is smaller it can cause one of the tiny infarcts that may not paralyse the nerves and muscles but will knock out part of the intellectual function of the brain.

Of course, atrial fibrillation, irregular beating of the pulse, is itself often the result of atherosclerosis of the blood vessels of the heart; arteries in the brain affected by high blood pressure are more likely to burst or become blocked, so these three types of problems (blood clots from atrial fibrillation, atherosclerosis, and high blood pressure) interact with one another as shown in Figure 4.2.

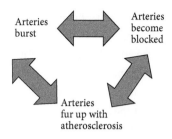

Figure 4.2 The three types of artery disasters.
Source the Optimal Ageing Programme.

Similarly, the risk factors for arterial disease overlap with one another. Several of these ideas were discussed in the previous chapters and overlap here. Though this time it is applied to arteries as opposed to just brain tissue.

Many of the twenty-first century health problems are the result of a combination of inactivity and diet. For example, type 2 diabetes is due to both reduced activity levels and increased calorie intake in most people. Similarly, hypercholesterolaemia, raised levels of cholesterol in the bloodstream, is also due to a combination of these two factors in most people. There are some people who have a genetic disorder which means that they have high levels of cholesterol no matter how active they are. Usually activity and diet are two sides of the coin, or like Yin and Yang, or interwoven like the warp and weft of Harris Tweed. Thus, we will consider diet and type 2 diabetes and raised levels of cholesterol in this chapter.

Raised levels of blood pressure occur not only as a result of obesity, but also from many other factors which we do not understand. Even lean people can have high blood pressure. So, for this reason we will consider blood pressure on its own, except to emphasize that keeping your weight down is a good way of preventing high blood pressure, and if high blood pressure has been diagnosed, of reducing the blood pressure. In summary, therefore, in this chapter we are going to consider several topics, but they do overlap and interrelate. When, however, a person develops one of these conditions they are often put on a pathway by their health service which makes it feel as if their condition, type 2 diabetes for example, is a separate condition, whereas it is part of a group of conditions that often occur together. This group of conditions has been given fancy names such as 'the metabolic syndrome'. From our point of view, we think the advice is very simple, namely:

- Maintain and increase your physical activity.
  - Reduce the risk of obesity.
- Rebalance your diet and take more activity.
  - Reduce your risk of type 2 diabetes.
  - Reduce your risk of hypercholesterolaemia
  - If you smoke, try stopping.
- If you have atrial fibrillation, make sure you get treatment to prevent blood clots forming.
- If you have had a TIA make sure you get treatment to reduce the risk of having a second TIA.

Rebalance your diet

There are two imbalances that increase the risk of dementia:

- The intake/expenditure imbalance.
- The dietary mix imbalance.

What is the evidence that diet reduces risk of dementia?

Studies using animal models have described the mechanisms through which certain dietary patterns can improve or harm brain health. Research on the impact of the Mediterranean diet, DASH diet (Dietary Approaches to Stop Hypertension) and the MIND diet (Mediterranean DASH Intervention for Neurodegenerative Delay) provides evidence on how diet can affect brain health. The research shows that a healthy diet is crucial to improve Brainability

Reduce the intake and increase the expenditure of energy

A healthy balance of energy intake from food and drink and energy expenditure from physical activity is required to maintain a healthy weight, which is a combination of strong healthy bones, adequate muscle development, and low levels of body fat. This weight is unique to everyone, due to the relative proportion of bone, muscle, and fat and is partly, but only partly, determined by genetics. One way to assess healthy weight in adults is to consider both height and weight. This measurement is known as body mass index (BMI). It is calculated by dividing the body weight in kilograms (kg) by the height in metres squared, that is multiplied by itself (m^2). For example, an individual who is 1.57 m (5'2") and weighs 54.5 kg (120 lb.), would have a BMI of 22. A BMI between 20–25 represents a 'healthy weight zone' which is associated with a lower occurrence of high blood pressure, diabetes, heart disease, and cancer. You can also determine your own BMI using one of the many charts you can find online.

Change the mix of your diet

Let's start with the good news; there is a growing consensus that what is commonly known as the Mediterranean diet, ticks all the boxes of essential nutrients for maintenance of optimal blood circulation in your brain. Few people would argue that people who live in Spain or Italy eat a miserable diet, so aim to eat more:

- Fruit and vegetables, why not seven a day rather than five?
- Protein from plants rather than animals, for example from nuts, peas, lentils, and chickpeas.
- Fish, especially fatty fish like tuna and mackerel.
- Chicken.

For many people not living on the Med this means a shift in many basic eating habits, such as shifting from red to white meat and substituting animal fats for olive oil. In addition, it is essential to avoid, or cut out completely if you can, high fat, high calorie temptations. These are almost always in shiny wrappers at the supermarket till or small shop counter, namely biscuits sweets, and chocolate. Refined white sugar should be avoided.

There is no strong evidence that any single chemical or vitamin can reduce the risk of dementia.

Support from family and friends

Once you have decided to change your diet, make small and measurable changes. These are easier to make and usually cause less difficulty. For example, try eating one more piece of fruit a day than you usually do. To help you identify your own barriers to changing your eating habits, think about the last few times you thought about changing your eating behaviour but did not follow through with it. Consider what held you back and write down your reasons. For each of your reasons, write a response that helps you reconsider your choice. Look at your list of reasons and responses whenever you are about to make a choice about what to eat.

You can change your food choices, but this requires overcoming barriers, so it is best to do it with friends and family involved. Usually we eat with friends and families and we are subject to their food choices. Talk to your family members and friends to see if any of them want to make a similar change or cheer you on as you change your food choices. Ask others how they manage to fit good nutrition into their lives.

Support in the community

Increasingly, communities are taking action to increase awareness of healthy eating and create environments to encourage healthy food choices. For example, many jurisdictions now require restaurants to identify in menus the number of calories within each food item. This is thought to help individuals to make better food choices.

Support from the health service

Sometimes your self-esteem holds you back from making healthy food choices. If this is an issue, counselling can help with issues of self-esteem. The success you feel from improving your eating habits may also improve your self-esteem. Bit by bit, you may begin to change the way you view yourself and your ability to change. Ask at your health centre for information in the first instance, then to get the name of someone who can help. Dietitians are few and far between, but most nurses in health centres know what the evidence is and how to communicate it.

Free high-quality systematic reviews of the evidence
  Cao, L., Tan, L., Wang, H.F., Jiang, T., Zhu, X.C., Lu, H., et al. (2016). Dietary patterns and risk of dementia: A systematic review and meta-analysis of cohort studies. *Molecular Neurobiology*, 53, 6144–6154.
  Global Council on Brain Health (2018). *Brain-Food GCBH Recommendations on Nourishing Your Brain Health.* Available at: www.GlobalCouncilOnBrainHealth.org doi: https://doi.org/10.26419/pia.00019.001
  Wu, S., Ding, Y., Wu, F., Li, R., Hou, J., & Mao, P. (2015). Omega-3 fatty acids intake and risks of dementia and Alzheimer's disease: A meta-analysis. *Neuroscience & Biobehavioral Reviews*, 48, 1–9.
  Zhang, Y., Chen, J., Qiu, J., Li, Y., Wang, J., & Jiao, J. (2016). Intakes of fish and polyunsaturated fatty acids and mild-to-severe cognitive impairment risks: A dose-response meta-analysis of 21 cohort studies. *American Journal of Clinical Nutrition*, 103, 330–340.

Keep your blood sugar low, avoid type 2 diabetes

Recent research has emphasized the importance of type 2 diabetes as a factor which increases the risk of dementia. The recent Lancet Commission on Dementia Prevention, Intervention and Care used experts from around the world to assemble systematically the best evidence and gave great emphasis to the importance of preventing type 2 diabetes and tackling it effectively if it develops (Livingston et al., 2017).

Type 2 diabetes (non-insulin dependent) is completely different from type 1 diabetes (insulin dependent), which is a disease of unknown cause, and type 2 can be both prevented and effectively managed. Not only are there effective medicines but, even more importantly, we now know that increasing physical activity, and therefore energy output, and decreasing energy intake can help to control type 2 diabetes and can indeed cure it. The word cure in this instance, is used appropriately. It is a condition resulting from our modern world, a world in which the amount of activity we must do has been progressively decreased and therefore the amount of energy we expend gets less and less each year. This, combined with the availability of food, particularly the availability of food that is high in calories and low in volume, is a contributing factor.

Why is type 2 diabetes a risk factor?

It may be that type 2 diabetes has a direct effect on the brain, but its main impact is on the blood supply. Type 2 diabetes increases the risk of atherosclerosis, the 'porridgy' type of material that builds up in the walls of arteries and blocks the blood supply either slowly or quickly when a clot forms. To keep your arteries healthy and therefore to keep the supply of oxygen plentiful it is essential to lower your risk of disease of the arteries. Preventing and managing type 2 diabetes is a key way of doing this.

How common is type 2 diabetes?

Type 2 diabetes is a common condition, often associated with being overweight or obese. Sometimes adults who are thin and active get diabetes and are told they have type 2 diabetes. However, there is increasing use of the term 'type 1 diabetes of adult onset', where something has obviously happened, perhaps an infection leading to an immune response that attacks the parts of the pancreas that produce insulin, thus causing a failure to control the level of sugar in the blood. Most people with type 2 diabetes develop it because they have had difficulty adapting to the low energy expenditure, high energy intake life typical of the twenty-first century.

How strong is the evidence that good type 2 diabetes control reduces the risk of dementia?

The evidence at present is clear that type 2 diabetes increases the risk of dementia. There is also evidence from population follow-up studies that improving the control of type 2 diabetes does reduce risk, but it may take more years for conclusive evidence based on systematic reviews of clinical trials to be produced. However, the link between type 2 diabetes and dementia risk, and the knowledge that type 2 diabetes affects the arteries is so strong that we can strongly advise the need to either prevent, control, or cure type 2 diabetes as one of the key steps in maintaining Brainability and reducing the risk of dementia (Biessels & Despa, 2018).

How can risk from type 2 diabetes be reduced?

Diabetes UK has advised that: 'diet and exercise can control type 2 diabetes and sometimes medication is needed too.' This quote emphasizes that an increase our activity and decreased energy intake should be utilized before medication. Modern medication is important, powerful, and based on good research. However, simply giving medication too quickly without advice, dietary support, or exercise will make people think that type 2 diabetes is a condition that is only treated by drugs. The main difference between type 1 and type 2 diabetes is that insulin is not usually required for people with type 2 diabetes. This approach is wrong, and you can change your food choices, but this requires overcoming barriers, so it is best to do it with friends and family involved. If you have type 2 diabetes it becomes even more important to increase activity and change to a Mediterranean or MIND diet.

What can you do to avoid type 2 diabetes?

The message is contained in our sections about increasing activity and rebalancing diet.

The modern environment is difficult and hazardous, particularly for people who are commuting and have a desk job, so you have to be aware of the dangers of the modern environment, dangers, for example, that lurk beside every checkout where calorie rich food packages are stacked high.

What sources of support are there to fight type 2 diabetes?

Friends and family support
When you share mealtimes with friends and family, make sure that they eat the same food. The low-calorie drinks that provide a new treatment for type 2 diabetes are not for everyone, except those with type 2 diabetes who want to both prevent and cure it. Exercise is also fundamental for diabetes management. Friends and family can make exercise easier by agreeing to exercise together. If you are a person with diabetes you should speak to your healthcare adviser, in order to find out what type of exercise will best suit your condition.

Community support
It is worthwhile joining Diabetes UK. As a member, you not only receive regular information, but also belong to a community of people with or caring for people with type 2 diabetes. Their website also allows the opportunity for exchanging ideas and support with other people.

Health service support
Your local health centre, primary care team, and practice nurse are well informed about type 2 diabetes. All of whom can give advice and support. The pharmacy in which you pick up your medication can also be helpful. Pharmacies play a leading role in the management of type 2 diabetes.

Free high-quality systematic reviews of the evidence
  Cheng, G., Huang, C., Deng, H., & Wang, H. (2012). Diabetes as a risk factor for dementia and mild cognitive impairment: A meta-analysis of longitudinal studies. *International Medicine*, J42, 484–484.
  Gudala, K., Bansal, D., Schifano, F., & Bhansali, A. (2013). Diabetes mellitus and risk of dementia: A meta-analysis of prospective observational studies. *Journal of Diabetes Investigation*, 4, 640–650.

Keep your cholesterol low

Cholesterol is essential for all body tissues to function properly. It is also a key component in fatty deposits and plaque that build up in arteries. Total blood cholesterol levels greater or equal to 5.2 mmol/L are considered a risk factor for cardiovascular disease but the risk of cholesterol is often linked to other risk factors and not just considered on its own. The debate about whether everyone over 75 should be offered statins is lively, with experts on both sides not yet in agreement. Cholesterol levels are lowered by taking statins, which also reduce the risk of strokes, heart attacks, and other cardiovascular diseases. We now know that any action that reduces the risk of stroke will reduce the risk of mini strokes or transient ischaemic attacks. The scientific evidence indicates that memory loss is not a side effect of taking statins (Schultz et al., (2018).

What is cholesterol?

Cholesterol is a fat-based substance found in the bloodstream and the body's cells. Essential for good health, cholesterol builds and repairs cells, protects nerve fibres, and is used to produce certain hormones and bile acids. Our body receives cholesterol from two sources: the liver produces it, and it is contained in foods such as meat, chicken, fish, eggs, and dairy products. You can lower your cholesterol by eating a healthy, balanced diet that's low in saturated fat. Exercising regularly, not smoking, and cutting down on alcohol also help to lower cholesterol (see Figure 4.3).

High cholesterol is a warning sign

In atherosclerosis, the walls of the arteries degenerate. This is caused by the accumulation of fatty deposits and inflammation in tissue, which leads to the restriction of blood circulation and blood clots. High levels of cholesterol are associated with this condition. Accumulation of fatty deposits on the walls of arteries are the principal cause of stroke, mini strokes, and other forms of cardiovascular system disease.

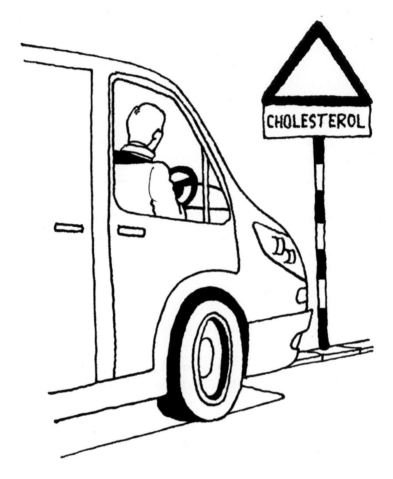

Figure 4.3 Take action to reduce high cholesterol as it also leads to dementia.
Source the Optimal Ageing Programme.

What are statins?

Statins were formerly known as HMG-CoA reductase inhibitors. Their purpose is to reduce cholesterol levels which then reduces the risk of strokes and mini strokes. These supplement the effects of other cholesterol lowering methods, such as low-fat diets and physical activity. Statins have greater cholesterol-lowering efficacy because once taken, they influence the interactions among molecules in the cells of arteries which create high levels of the types of cholesterol and fatty acids that cause arterial disease.

How strong is the evidence that lowering cholesterol can reduce the risk of dementia?

Total cholesterol levels greatly increase cardiovascular and total mortality. The association between cholesterol and disease is mostly from studies more focused on younger subjects. However, because cardiovascular disease is relatively rare in the younger population, the impact of high cholesterol on health is still stronger in older people. When cholesterol moves through our blood, it joins up with proteins to make molecules known as lipoproteins. 'Bad' cholesterol, or low-density lipoproteins (LDL), can build up on the walls of blood vessels, blocking and damaging arteries. This can eventually cause heart disease and strokes. But there's also 'good' cholesterol, high-density lipoproteins (HDL), which clear away the dangerous type of cholesterol. Although LDL is the one to worry about, getting accurate readings of both kinds is essential. High levels of 'bad' cholesterol and low levels of 'good' cholesterol indicate a higher risk of stroke, heart disease, and vascular dementia as Collins et al. demonstrated.

Blood cholesterol levels are reported as milligrams per decilitre (e.g. 220 mg/dL) or millimoles per litre (e.g. 5.20 mmol/L). After its first year of being taken, statin therapy reduces the risk of strokes, heart attacks, coronary deaths, and the need for coronary artery surgery or stent procedures, by about one-quarter for each mmol/L reduction in LDL cholesterol. Lowering LDL cholesterol by 2 mmol/L (77 mg/dL) can be achieved with an effective low-cost statin regimen (such as a 40 mg atorvastatin daily). Over five years, 10,000 patients taking statin would typically prevent major vascular events from occurring in about 1000 patients who had pre-existing vascular disease. It also prevents them from occurring in 500 patients who are at increased risk but have not yet had a vascular event. Statin therapy has been shown to reduce vascular disease risk during each year it continues to be taken, so greater benefits would accrue with more prolonged therapy, with the benefits persisting long term.

Misinformation about statins' effect on memory and other aspects of cognition

The US Food and Drug Administration (FDA) updated its safety information for statins in 2017. The new information no longer includes memory loss, forgetfulness, and confusion as possible risks, or side effects of taking statins. While statin users have reported memory loss to the FDA, studies have not found evidence to support these claims. Despite information on the Internet and numerous publications about side effects of statins, systematic reviews of available evidence from randomized trials have not found evidence of any adverse effects of exposure to statin therapy on a wide range of different cognitive measures (Schultz et al., 2018).

The benefits of statins are well established and are considered to outweigh the risk of side effects in most people taking statins. The efficacy and safety of statins has been studied in several large trials which show that they can lower the level of cholesterol in the blood, reduce cardiovascular disease, and save lives. Trials have also shown that medically significant side effects are rare. Consequently, given the lack of evidence of adverse effects of statin therapy on memory or cognition, it is now appropriate for regulatory authorities to consider removing them from drug labels as potential side effects. This will ensure that patients are not inappropriately deterred from using statin therapy. Changing the false information circulating online, however, continues to be challenging.

What can you do to keep cholesterol as low as possible?

Taking statins is not by itself the answer to us to continuing to live unhealthily, but more of an added treatment, together with the other interventions. We need to look after ourselves by not smoking or drinking heavily and exercising more, in addition to taking statins. It is important that we do not think of statins as the answer to everything.

Free high-quality systematic reviews of the evidence
Anstey, K.J., Ashby-Mitchell, K., & Peters, R. (2017). Updating the evidence on the association between serum cholesterol and risk of late-life dementia: Review and meta-analysis. *Journal of Alzheimer's Disease*, 56, 215–228.
Richardson, K., Schoen, M., French, B., Umscheid, C.A., Mitchell, M.D., Arnold, S.E., et al., (2013). Statins and cognitive function: A systematic review. *Annals Internal Medicine*, 159, 688–697.

Keep your blood pressure low

The higher your blood pressure the greater the risk of brain damage either from a stroke or from mini strokes. High blood pressure is a condition of unknown cause, but the risk of high blood pressure is increased by inactivity and obesity. Reducing blood pressure reduces the risk of dementia. Since most people with high blood pressure have no specific warning signs or symptoms, it is important to have blood pressure checked regularly.

What is the right blood pressure?

Blood pressure is determined by the power of the heart which pumps blood out and the resistance of the blood vessels. The resistance of the blood vessels is the key factor. Blood flows through the blood vessels continuously, with the pressure at its highest when the heart beats and lowest when the heart is filling again. This means that the pressure is expressed as two numbers. The highest pressure is called the systolic pressure and the lowest the diastolic pressure. These pressure levels are expressed in this way 145/82 or 132/68. Doctors and nurses sometimes call it '145 over 82' or '132 over 68'. The actual measurements are in millimetres of mercury, written in your notes as mm Hg (from the Latin *hydrargyrum*, meaning liquid silver). That was the way pressure was measured in old-fashioned sphygmomanometers, but it is usually done now by an electric motor pumping air into a cuff wrapped round the arm. You can measure this yourself by using a 'sphyg', an automated blood pressure measuring device available at any pharmacy. It is good to do this if you are being treated for blood pressure to make sure that the treatment is right for you.

There is debate about the right level of blood pressure but there is now a view that we should aim for blood pressure less than 120 over 70 (120/70). This should be your target, particularly if there are other risk factors for dementia. The *Journal of the American Medical Association* selected the paper describing the research supporting the benefits of lowering blood pressure to 120 in people over 75 on Hogmanay 2019 as one of their top ten papers of the decade (Williamson et al., 2016).

How does high blood pressure lead to dementia?

Whilst the human brain comprises only about 2.5% of the body's weight, it receives almost 15% of the blood flow from the heart and uses as much as 25% of the body's total oxygen consumption. Any reduction or interruption of this flow can cause strokes or mini strokes, which damage brain tissue and cause or contribute to dementia. It is important to maintain the ideal pressure within the arteries, and the arterioles (the small vessels in the brain). The arteries and arterioles get the blood to where it is needed, but it is in the smallest vessels in the brain tissue, the capillaries, where the oxygenated blood coming from the lungs via the heart passes into the brain. There are as many as four hundred miles of these blood vessels in the brain and they cover a surface area the size of a tennis court. Blood pressure that is too high adversely affects the flow of blood to the brain (see Figure 4.4). At very high levels this predisposes to major life-threatening strokes, as well as contributing to mini strokes, some of which are called 'silent strokes'.

If a blood vessel develops a leak (called a haemorrhagic stroke) the supply of oxygen to the brain from that artery is diminished. Silent

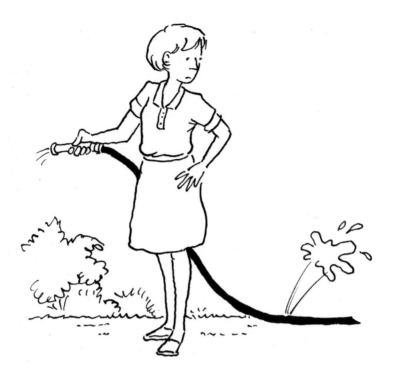

Figure 4.4 Strokes occur when there is a temporary drop in blood supply to the brain.
Source the Optimal Ageing Programme.

strokes are small strokes that affect parts of the brain that do not control movement and thus go unnoticed. Mini strokes or TIAs occur when there is a temporary drop in the blood supply to the brain, leading to temporary stroke-like symptoms. These are signs that the blood supply to the brain is not in good order and therefore needs special attention, which we will discuss later.

High blood pressure, sometimes called hypertension, is a common treatable 'silent' condition, as it can often cause no symptoms for years. It has predisposing causes, such as kidney disease, but in most people it has no obvious predisposing cause. This is sometimes referred to by an old-fashioned term 'essential hypertension'. Blood pressure that is too high causes systemic and widespread damage to the walls of arteries.

Healthy arteries are flexible, strong, and elastic, with a smooth inner lining that blood flows through freely, supplying vital organs and tissues with adequate nutrients and oxygen. If you have high blood pressure then the increased pressure in your arteries can gradually cause a variety of problems, including damage to the cells lining your arteries. This triggers a series of events that make artery walls thick and stiff. Fats from your diet enter your bloodstream, pass through the damaged cells, and collect in clumps on the vessel walls, in the condition known as atherosclerosis. All these changes increase the risk of coronary heart disease when they occur in the arteries supplying the muscular wall of the heart, causing heart attacks and different types of strokes. Strokes are the second most common cause of death. Most are caused by clots blocking the blood vessels (ischaemic strokes), in most of the remainder of cases, the damaged blood vessel walls leak and cause a bleed into the brain tissue.

Most of the different types of dementia, including specific conditions, like Alzheimer's disease, have a vascular component. This means that problems with the blood vessels in the brain are either the main cause of the dementia or are a significant contributory factor. It is thus important to try to find out if you have a level of blood pressure that should be lowered to reduce your risk of dementia. It is identifiable and treatable. Even more encouragingly, if we treat it, not only is the risk of developing dementia reduced, but the disease progression of established dementia is slowed. As a bonus, reducing blood pressure also reduces damage to our heart and kidneys, thus reducing the chance of developing heart failure, heart attacks, and abnormalities of heart rhythm, such as atrial fibrillation.

How strong is the evidence about reducing blood pressure to reduce the risk of dementia?

According to the *World Alzheimer Report 2014* (Wortmann, 2015), multiple studies following large groups of people for 15–40 years, demonstrated that individuals who had high blood pressure in mid-life (characterized as people aged around 40–64) were more likely to develop dementia in later life. However, the benefits of controlling blood pressure continue in later age groups and the evidence about the benefits of reducing blood pressure after the age of 65 is increasing every year. We know that as many as a third of people who experience strokes, develop dementia in the first year after. The number who then exhibit symptoms of dementia increases in subsequent years (Wortmann, 2015).

If you have developed high blood pressure, you are not alone; as many as one in three adults develop high blood pressure at some point in their lives in the UK. Out of these sixteen million people, seven million people are living with undiagnosed high blood pressure, not knowing they are at risk. The only way to know whether you have high blood pressure is to have it measured. Anyone over the age of 40 should have it checked regularly, certainly every few years at least. Once it is diagnosed, there are many ways it can be treated both with lifestyle modification and the use of drugs. Having high blood pressure does not cause any discomfort and some people find it difficult to stick to their treatment plans, but it is worthwhile to persevere as you can reduce your risks of developing dementia. We also know that even if you do not have high blood pressure, making some simple lifestyle changes may help prevent you developing it in the future (Sharp et al., 2011).

How can blood pressure be reduced?

Having a family history of high blood pressure, is a well-known risk factor and there is nothing we can do to alter who our parents are. We can, however, take more care to reduce modifiable risk factors, because acting early can affect our chances of developing high blood pressure in the future. Everyone can reduce the risk of developing strokes and dementia if we manage our modifiable risk factors such as:

- Being overweight. The more you weigh the more blood you need to supply oxygen and nutrients to your tissues. As the volume of blood circulated through your blood vessels increases, so does the pressure on your artery walls. Obesity also predisposes to type 2 diabetes.

- Using tobacco. Smoking damages the lining of your artery walls. This can cause your arteries to narrow, increasing your blood pressure. Second-hand smoke also can increase your blood pressure.
- Having too much salt in your diet. Too much salt in the diet can cause fluid retention, which leads to an increase in blood pressure.
- Drinking too much alcohol. Over time, heavy drinking can damage both your heart and your brain.
- Not doing enough exercise. In addition to the positive effect of exercise on our arteries and the beneficial effects of exercise on weight, people who are inactive tend to have higher blood pressure.

However old you are it is never too late to start to manage your risk better. Can you manage all your risk factors all at once? Can you change your behaviour overnight? Can you turn the clock back and look ten years younger, have more vigour, fun, and purpose? The answer to all these questions is 'yes'. But we are not all the same, we do not all have the same make-up or motivation, so start by taking small steps and building on it. Make a single change in your life and when comfortable with it, make another. It will get easier with each change and you will feel better for it. Through reading this book, you now know that many of these predisposing conditions cause no outward signs for a while and the quicker you start to manage them, the greater the chances of you managing your risks better.

Am I on the right track with my blood pressure?

Everyone over 60 should know their blood pressure. You can now purchase the equipment to measure blood pressure accurately. This can be done in every health centre and everyone aged 40 plus should be offered a health check every five years. The only people who are not offered a health check every five years, are those who are already getting checked regularly due to high blood pressure or heart disease. Everyone should know their blood pressure. Everyone should aim to have a blood pressure less than 140 over 80, if you have any other risk factors you should aim for 130 over 70. The new guidelines from the American Heart Association and the American College of Cardiology, released in

November 2017, lowered the threshold for diagnosing high blood pressure from 140/90 to 130/80. This means that nearly half of the population will be considered as having high blood pressure. That is not to say that half the population should take medication for high blood pressure, because for many the pressure can be lowered by reducing weight and increasing activity.

What sources of support are there to lower blood pressure?

Support from friends and family

Friends and family need to know that high blood pressure is symptomless. They can also be of assistance in reminding you to have your blood pressure taken each time you visit the health centre, or assist you with putting on the cuff of your 'sphyg', your automated blood pressure measuring device, if you find this difficult to do on your own. Your pharmacist can advise which one is right for you.

Support from the community

Research shows that meeting with other people with high blood pressure can help reduce blood pressure. The main benefit is the activities that are available both for weight reduction and increased activity. Weight clubs are effective and joining a gym or fitness centre or swimming at the local pool are also effective means of blood pressure reduction.

Support from the health service

The key professional support comes from the staff in your health centre, particularly the practice nurse. Pharmacists also know a lot about blood pressure and can help people find the right mix of drugs to help get their blood pressure down below the key level that is right for them.

Correct measurement of blood pressure

It is sensible to buy an automated blood pressure measuring device and measure your pressure once a month following the steps below:

- Don't exercise or consume caffeine within 30 minutes.
- Empty your bladder.
- Sit in a chair with your feet flat on the ground and legs uncrossed, with your back supported for five minutes.
- Roll up your sleeve so the blood pressure cuff rests on bare skin.
- Your arm should be supported on a table or a desk.

See Figure 4.5.

If your blood pressure appears high, your physician or pharmacist or nurse should take a reading in both arms. The next time you visit, the reading should be from the arm that showed the higher pressure. There

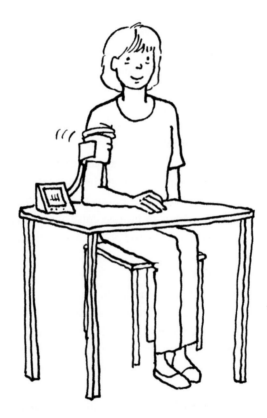

Figure 4.5 Blood pressure is best measured when sitting quietly and not talking with someone.
Source the Optimal Ageing Programme.

is no single number that determines your blood pressure, it can vary throughout the day and be influenced by something as simple as being approached by a well-meaning nurse carrying a blood pressure cuff. The diagnosis of high blood pressure requires at least two readings on separate occasions.

Free high-quality systematic reviews of the evidence
Sharp, S.I., Aarsland, D., Day, S., & Sonnesyn, H. (2011). Alzheimer's Society Vascular Dementia Systematic Review Group.
Ballard, C. (2011) Hypertension is a potential risk factor for vascular dementia: Systematic review. *International Journal of Geriatric Psychiatry*, 26, 661–669.
Hughes, T.M. & Sink, K.M. (2016). Hypertension and its role in cognitive function: Current evidence and challenges for the future. *American Journal of Hypertension*, 29(2), 149–157. doi: 10.1093/ajh/hpv180.

Stop smoking—you can do it

No matter how many times you have tried and failed, try again, using any help or support available. Overwhelming research evidence shows that inhaling cigarette smoke, your own or someone else's, increases your risk of many diseases and premature death. Smoking exposes people several times a day to chemicals which cause cancer, cardiovascular disease, and dementia. Among the many reasons that smokers do not quit is that smoking is an addiction. When a person stops smoking, they may experience physical and psychological symptoms that are not pleasant. Smoking is widespread throughout our culture. However, while at one time the social image of smokers was glamorous, smoking is less socially acceptable now. The recognition of the harmful effects of smoking has convinced many people to quit. Smoking cessation support can be provided by friends and family, and anti-smoking actions taken by businesses and governments. Within the health service, drugs that assist with reducing the chemical dependency created by smoking can be prescribed.

What is the evidence about the risk of dementia from smoking?

Much of the early concern about cigarette smoking 50 years ago focused on the increased risk of cancer. In the last 20 years it has become clear that smoking is also a major risk for heart disease. Even more recently, the effects of smoking on all the blood vessels of the body have been appreciated. The principal means by which smoking causes heart disease is by narrowing the arteries of the heart, not by affecting the heart directly. It is no surprise, therefore, that cigarette smoking has now been shown to increase the risk of dementia through its effect on the arteries that carry oxygen rich blood to the brain (Zhong et al., 2015). When an artery is affected by atherosclerosis it is at increased risk of either blocking off completely, thus depriving the part of the brain it supplies of oxygen, or bursting, which also cuts off the supply of oxygen and causes damage to brain tissue from the blood that has leaked out.

Creating stigma towards smoking through advertising

Cigarette advertising previously promoted a hazardous product, so the case was made for restricting advertising of cigarettes. Alarmed by the damage to human health caused by tobacco smoking, public authorities gradually transformed the public image of cigarettes from symbols of sophistication into objects of danger. Many countries require packaging that alerts smokers to the dangers of the 'cancer sticks' they are purchasing, and many packs carry health warnings, including the increased risk of dementia.

In some countries, such as Australia, images of the grievous bodily harm caused by prolonged exposure to tobacco smoke must be printed on cigarette cartons. These images are designed to discourage smoking and make plain the damage it causes. Campaigns against smoking have also emphasized the dangers to third parties, and children when they inhale second-hand smoke (see Figure 4.6).

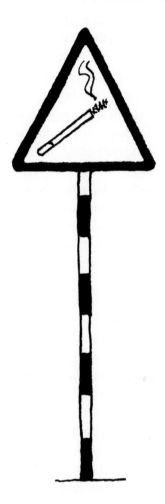

Figure 4.6 Take action to stop smoking.
Source the Optimal Ageing Programme.

How can you reduce your risk from smoking?

No matter how often you have tried and failed, try again, this time focused on the benefits in terms of a reduced risk of dementia. For example, look at NHS Choices online, or just type 'stop smoking' into a search engine to find advice on smoking. You can also contact your local health centre for a link to a service that can provide support.

Find out if you have atrial fibrillation and get treatment

Atrial fibrillation is a treatable condition that can cause both strokes and dementia, so it is important for it to be diagnosed and treated. Research shows a consistent association between atrial fibrillation and dementia. It is likely that several different factors combine to cause dementia in atrial fibrillation patients. Both atrial fibrillation and dementia share common risks, including smoking, high blood pressure, inactive lifestyle, and poor diet, each of these may be targets of early prevention strategies to reduce risk. Self-care of atrial fibrillation begins with an understanding of the treatment goal and actions to take if the treatment goal is not met or if adverse effects of treatment occur. Assessment of heart rate and rhythm is an important aspect of self-monitoring the response to treatment.

How does atrial fibrillation increase the risk of dementia?

Atrial fibrillation is a condition where the heart beats irregularly, allowing small blood clots to form in the heart. These can then break off and be carried in the bloodstream to the brain, where they can cause strokes or mini strokes. Atrial fibrillation is caused by a variety of factors, including high blood pressure and damage to the heart through atherosclerosis of the arteries. Silent strokes are mini strokes that affect parts of the brain which are not associated with movement and thus, again, often go unnoticed because they do not cause any obvious signs such as weakness of a leg. Mini strokes or TIAs occur when there is a temporary drop in the blood supply to the brain, leading to temporary stroke-like symptoms. Atrial fibrillation is a significant cause of strokes, mini strokes, and vascular dementia. People with atrial fibrillation are five times more likely to develop a stroke and the association between the two conditions is well understood and uncontroversial. Atrial fibrillation is a condition that does not require fancy equipment to diagnose. An 'irregularly irregular pulse' characterizes it. Normally the pulse is regular both in rhythm and in its strength, determined by the volume of blood flowing through the artery. In atrial fibrillation, the pulse tends to be fast and is irregular. Also, the volume varies, so some pulsations may be easy to feel when the amount of blood flowing is high, whereas others may be more difficult to feel as the blood flow may be reduced. So, not only is the rhythm irregular but also the volume often changes from beat to beat.

How strong is the evidence that controlling atrial fibrillation reduces the risk of dementia?

We know that as many as a third of people who develop strokes go on to develop dementia in the first year after a stroke and the number who then show symptoms of dementia increases in subsequent years. The evidence around the benefits of controlling atrial fibrillation to reduce the risk of dementia is strong (Kwok et al., 2011; Kalantarian et al., 2013).

What can you do about atrial fibrillation?

It is important to identify atrial fibrillation. It is easily identifiable and treatable. Even more encouragingly, if we treat it, the risk of developing dementia reduces, and disease progression is delayed if it has already started to develop.

How can you tell if you have atrial fibrillation?

Check your own pulse regularly. Atrial fibrillation occurs more frequently as we grow older and if we have high blood pressure. Some medical conditions also increase the chance of developing it. These conditions include heart problems such as coronary heart disease or disease of the heart's valves. It can also be caused by an overactive thyroid gland, lung infections like pneumonia, or a blood clot in the lung called a pulmonary embolism. Drinking too much alcohol or caffeine, taking illegal drugs, such as cocaine or amphetamines, or smoking can also trigger atrial fibrillation.

Importance of the health service to support those with atrial fibrillation

If you have atrial fibrillation, you will usually need treatment to control the condition and reduce your risk of stroke. This may involve taking some drugs called antiarrhythmics which make your heart beat more regularly, as well as slowing your heart rate. You may also be given anti-coagulants to reduce the chances of developing small clots. There are different types of anticoagulants and the choice of which to use depends on a more thorough examination and the medical history of the patient.

Free high-quality systematic reviews of the evidence

Kalantarian, S., Stern, T.A., Mansour, M., & Ruskin, J.N. (2013). Cognitive impairment associated with atrial fibrillation: A meta-analysis. *Annals of Internal Medicine*, 158, 338–346.

De Silva, R.M.F.L., Miranda, C.M., Liu, T., Tse, G., PRever L. (2019). Atrial fibrillation and risk of dementia: Epidemiology, mechanisms, and effect of anticoagulation. *Frontiers in Neuroscience*, 13, 18. doi:

If you have had a TIA, act

A TIA is a blockage in a small blood vessel in the brain which does not leave permanent damage to the part of the brain that control muscles and movement. It indicates a high risk of vascular dementia and the need for effective action to improve Brainability and reduce the risk of a stroke or vascular dementia. Everyone can identify a stroke because its effects are obvious: paralysis, usually of one side of the body. The paralysis occurs on the opposite side to the part of the brain in which a major blood vessel has been blocked or has burst. In the last 20 years it has also been noted that small arteries can become blocked. Sometimes this affects the muscles, causing facial weakness, but it always lasts less than 24 hours. This is a TIA. It is known that these also occur in the parts of the brain which control memory as well as parts of the brain that control the muscles, so they can be the first indication of vascular dementia. The risk of second and subsequent TIAs can be reduced.

How strong is the evidence about the benefits of responding to the challenge of a TIA?

It is only recently that TIAs have been recognized as an important clinical problem. The evidence for this emerged as the result of a development of a new technique for imaging of the brain called MRI. Before this, the only way to see what was happening in the brain in the blood vessels was to inject an opaque dye into the blood vessels. This was an unpleasant and risky procedure that only showed large blockages. With the development of MRI our ability to see what is happening in the brain has been dramatically improved. TIAs appear as white specs on the black substance of the brain. Some people develop what looks like a snowstorm, in these cases it represents vascular dementia. There is no doubt that having a TIA is a risk factor for having a major stroke and it is a risk factor for vascular dementia. It is difficult to do major trials, partly because it would now be unethical not to respond effectively and swiftly, but in our judgement the evidence is strong.

How can the risk be reduced?

The first step is to recognize when someone is having a TIA. The main stroke symptoms can be remembered with the acronym FAST:

- *Face*—the face may have dropped on one side, the person may not be able to smile, or their mouth or eye may have drooped.
- *Arms*—the person with suspected stroke may not be able to lift both arms and keep them there because of weakness or numbness in one arm.
- *Speech*—their speech may be slurred or garbled, or the person may not be able to talk at all despite appearing to be awake; they may also have problems understanding what you're saying to them.

- *Time*—dial your emergency number immediately if you notice any of these signs or symptoms.

The signs and symptoms of a stroke vary from person to person, but usually begin suddenly. As different parts of the brain control different parts of the body, the symptoms depend on the part of the brain affected and the extent of the damage. Response should be rapid. When a TIA occurs, there is a high risk of stroke during the following two weeks. Many of the measures to reduce the impact of TIAs on the brain are the same as the measures we described to reduce the vascular risk, but they need to be applied even more enthusiastically. If you or someone you care for has a TIA it is vitally important not just to control the blood pressure, but to bring the blood pressure down under 130/70.

Who is there to help?

As always, the primary care team is of vital importance, but the diagnosis requires hospital imaging and there is often a team linked to the stroke team with a special interest in getting the right treatment started for someone who has had one TIA to reduce the risk of a stroke and vascular dementia. The key issue therefore is prompt action.

Watch this space: Developments for which there is not yet evidence of effectiveness

Action against disease of the vascular system has two main strategies. The first is a medical strategy which focuses on diagnosing people at high risk and then treating them, for example with statins or drugs to lower blood pressure. The second approach is to try to change the risk profile of the whole population, for example by reducing salt in the diet to reduce the blood pressure of everyone. The high-risk approach identifies individuals who will benefit from education, psychological support, and medication. However, a large number of 'low-risk' people (having a level of risk at which drug treatment is not judged to be economically worthwhile), will have a heart attack or a stroke or develop dementia. They are at lower risk

---

Box 4.1 Free high-quality systematic reviews of the evidence

Georgakis, M.K., Duering, M., Wardlaw, J.M., & Dichgans, M. (2019). WMH and long-term outcomes in ischemic stroke: A systematic review and meta-analysis. *Neurology*, 92(12), e1298-e1308. doi: 10.1212/WNL.0000000000007142. Epub 15 Feb. 2019.

---

but there are so many of them that the total number affected is large, so we will see an increased focus on population health measures to change diet and promote activity.

The possible metformin bonus

One interesting focus of research at present is on the commonly prescribed drug for type 2 diabetes, metformin, which might have a direct effect on the ageing process. It is reported in the Scientific American's eBook *New Science of Healthy Aging*, that this possibility was observed by some researchers by chance. When looking at the results of a diabetes project, they found that older people who were taking metformin were living 18% longer than people who were like them in every other way but did not have diabetes and were not taking metformin. It is unclear how metformin might affect ageing, but there is now a randomized controlled trial of metformin to test whether metformin can slow down ageing. The trial is called Targeting Aging Metformin (because researchers choose a sexy acronym before making up the name of the trial) (see Box 4.1).

References

Ballard C. (2011). Hypertension is a potential risk factor for vascular dementia: systematic review. *International Journal of Geriatric Psychiatry*, 26, 661–669.

Biessels, G.J. & Despa, F. (2018). Cognitive decline and dementia in diabetes: Mechanisms and clinical implications. *Nature Reviews Endocrinology*, 10, 591–604.

Collins, R., Reith R., Emberson, J., Armitage, J., Baigent C., Blackwell L., et al. (2016). Interpretation of the evidence for the efficacy and safety of statin therapy. *Lancet*, 388(10059), 2532–2561.

Kalantarian, S., Stern T.A., Mansour M., Ruskin J.N. (2013). Cognitive impairment associated with atrial fibrillation: A meta-analysis. *Annals of Internal Medicine*, 158, 338–346.

Kwok, C.S., Loke Y.K., Hale R., Potter J.F., Mynt P.K. (2011). Atrial fibrillation and incidence of dementia: a systematic review and meta-analysis. *Neurology*, 10, 914–922.

Livingston, G., Sommerlad A., Orgeta V., Costafreda S.G., Huntley J., Ames D. (2017). The Lancet Commission on 'Dementia prevention, intervention, and care'. *Lancet*, 390, 2673–2734.

Prnice, M., Wimo, A., Guerchet, M., Ali, G., Wu. Y. (2015). World Alzheimer report 2014: Dementia and risk reduction. *Alzheimer's & Dementia*, 7S_Part_18, 837.

Schultz, B.G., Patten, D.K., Berlau, D.J. (2018). The role of statins in both cognitive impairment and protection against dementia: a tale of two mechanisms. *Translational Neurodegeneration*, 7, 5.

Williamson, J.D., Supiano, M.A., Applegate, W.B., Berlowitz, D.R., Campbell, R.C., Chertow, G.M. (2016). Intensive vs standard blood pressure control and cardiovascular disease outcomes in adults aged ≥75 years: A randomized clinical trial. *Journal of American Medical Association*, 24, 2673.

Zhong, G., Wang, Y., Zhang, Y., Guo, J., Zhao, Y. (2015). Smoking is associated with an increased risk of dementia: A meta-analysis of prospective cohort studies with investigation of potential effect modifiers. *PLoS ONE*, 3, e0118333.

5

Increase Your Ability to Interact with People and Ideas

When we were students studying the structure and function of the human body, we found that the brain was both complex and simple to understand. The structure and function of the brain was complex, with various parts having peculiar names, like 'hippocampus'. However, there was one simple fact that was helpful. The brain we were born with, we were told, did not grow or develop. It could, and probably would, be damaged by disease but the nerve cells or neurons would not develop or change. They would just gradually reduce in number.

That teaching was wrong. The brain is an organ that can grow and develop. The term that has entered research and education about the brain is plasticity, neuroplasticity specifically. Plastic implies a material that is hard and strong and shiny, the great advantage of which is that you can change its form easily. Through the application of heat, plastic can bend or transform from a toy car to a spoon or vice versa. The brain is like plastic. Neuroplasticity means that the brain can develop throughout life. New networks of nerve cells develop as a result of learning. The nervous system is not a set of electric cables connecting the brain to a foot, hand, or eye. It is better to think of it as a set of networks, like a train network which people can use in a million ways. New routes can be discovered by people reaching their seventies and beyond.

When you learn a new skill, like how to dance the tango, additional nerve cells are produced to help you carry out the steps. The existing neurons form new connections to other existing neurons, creating new networks. The brain acts like an ant colony. When ants face a challenge, they communicate with each another until a solution emerges. The

Increase your Brainability—and Reduce your Risk of Dementia. Charles Alessi, Larry W. Chambers, and Muir Gray, Oxford University Press. © Oxford University Press 2021. DOI: 10.1093/oso/9780198860341.003.0005

queen does not tell them what to do as that is not her job; the workers solve the problem on their own. Once the colony has solved a problem, they know how to solve that same problem more quickly next time. Learning comes about through the creation of neural networks and new research demonstrates that there is no upper age limit for network formation. People who have been diagnosed with dementia also need continuing opportunities to form new networks, learn, and develop. There are three ways in which this aspect of Brainability can be improved:

- By learning new skills, preferably by engaging in purposeful work.
- By maintaining and increasing contact and interaction with other people.
- By maintaining hearing and vision to keep receiving stimulation.

Learning new skills

Neuroplasticity, also known as brain or neural plasticity, is the brain's ability to create new connections throughout the length of an individual's life. It is no longer thought that the brain only develops during early childhood and remains unchanged throughout adult life, into old age. There is even evidence that new brain cells can develop, a process called neurogenesis.

Any intellectual activity is better than inactivity, the more challenging the better. Cryptic crosswords are better than ordinary crosswords and learning a language or musical instrument is better than both. However, if the intellectual activity involves more time sitting at a desk or screen, it may increase the risk of dementia by reducing your time spent being physically active. It is important to give priority to intellectual activity that involves engagement with other people, playing bridge is better than sitting on your own playing computer games. The best form of activity is one that gets you involved and engaging with other people, helping young children learn how to read, for example. Volunteering ticks all the boxes, particularly because it is often difficult and challenging, so being on the bridge club committee is even better than playing bridge (particularly if the members are a difficult bunch).

What is meant by increased intellectual activity?

Lifelong intellectual activity prevents intellectual decline. As with physical ability, the higher your ability when you start to decline the better. Usually the people who were lucky enough to be born into a family that valued education and had the money to support it start from a higher point, as shown in Figure 5.1.

Those people with higher education may be more highly motivated to pursue intellectual stimulation throughout their life. However, whatever your opportunities were early in life, it is never too late to increase your knowledge, skills, and learning. As with physical ability, most people decline more quickly due to more than just ageing. There is what can be considered 'fitness gap analogous' to the physical ability fitness gap that gets wider with age. As with loss of physical fitness, the gap can be narrowed by increased activity at any age, as shown in Figure 5.2.

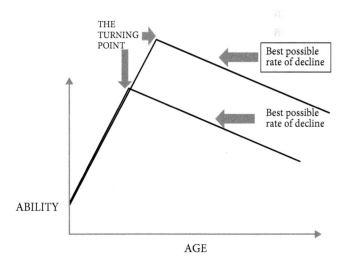

Figure 5.1 The impact of education on the level of ability.
Source the Optimal Ageing Programme.

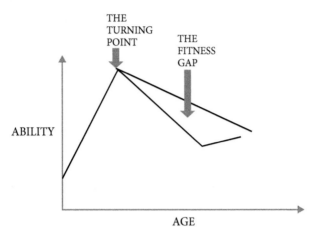

Figure 5.2 Closing the ability gap.
Source the Optimal Ageing Programme.

What happens to our intellectual activity as we age?

Reduction in intellectual abilities appears to be a part of normal ageing. Aspects of intellectual or cognitive abilities such as memory, reasoning, processing speed, and verbal ability decline at the same speed. However, there is evidence that reasoning and speed of processing can be improved through training. Older adults can, and do, successfully use compensatory approaches to offset intellectual decline, due to knowledge, skills, and experience that young adults may not have. People acquire 'assets', to use the term made popular by Lynda Gratton and Andrew Scott in their book *The 100-Year Life*. Older people may make better decisions, specifically the kind that require reflection and experience. The authors place a welcome emphasis on the 'assets' people acquire as they live longer and not on the losses which are usually the focus of writing on ageing. By 'assets' they are not referring to financial assets, but the psychological and social assets which they classify as being of three sorts:

1. The first category of intangibles is productive assets. These are the assets that help an individual become productive and successful at work and should therefore boost their income. Obviously, skills and

knowledge will be a major component of this category, but there is much else as well.

2. The second category is vitality assets. Broadly, these capture mental and physical health and well-being. Included here are friendship, positive family relationships and partnerships, as well as personal fitness and health.

3. The final category is transformational assets. Across a 100-year life, people will experience great change and many transitions. These transformational assets refer to their self-knowledge, their capacity to reach out into diverse networks and their openness to new experiences.

(Gratton & Scott, 2016)

Ageing populations are extremely heterogeneous, with older adults varying in ability due to differences in genetics and experiences over their lifespans (see Figure 5.3).

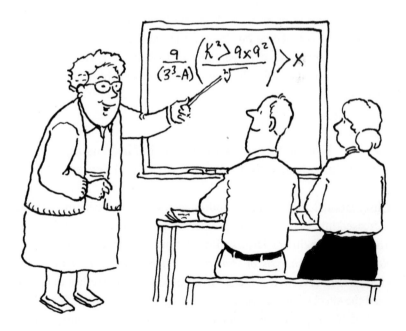

Figure 5.3 Never make assumptions on the basis of age or appearance.
Source the Optimal Ageing Programme.

It is wise not to make assumptions based on someone's chronological age

Today's older adults did not grow up using computers and therefore would not be expected to be as fluent with computer and Internet use. However, groups differ in their intellectual abilities and even individuals in the same age group differ from each other. People of any given age differ from one another in as many ways as they are similar. In the short term, individuals will differ from time to time because of fatigue, acute illness, distractions, and attention lapses. In the long term, there are ups and downs in intellectual abilities throughout an individual's life. Studies of whole populations reveal that people's intellectual abilities differ at different ages, not only because of ageing.

Conditions that affect intellectual abilities such as cardiovascular diseases, diabetes, and dementia, increase with age. It is important to emphasize that just because a disease increases in prevalence as we get older, this does not mean ageing causes the disease. Often the reason common diseases increase with age, is that people have been exposed to the risk factors for longer, for example they have been smoking or eating a diet that raises the risk of type 2 diabetes for longer. Sensory decline in seeing and hearing increases with age, these may be due to ageing rather than to environmental or lifestyle issues, but improvement is almost always possible.

How strong is the evidence that increasing intellectual activity reduces the risk of dementia?

Observational studies and a randomized, controlled trial indicate that increased intellectual activity prevents cognitive decline and dementia. The 2014 Alzheimer's Disease International report on *Dementia Risk Reduction: An Analysis of Protective and Modifiable Factors* (Pender et al., 2014), reviewed evidence from observational studies that measured the effect of education on developing dementia later in life. The review of 30 cohort studies concluded that there was a definite protective effect of higher education in high-income countries. It also showed that no one should assume that a poor education in their youth cannot reduce their risk of dementia by increasing intellectual activity. Remember that individuals with less of an education may simply perform worse on neuropsychological tests, even though they have the same level of intelligence. The apparent relationship between education and dementia may be because of the better educated person's ability to perform better on the tests.

The 2014 Alzheimer's Disease International report also reviewed evidence from population studies that measured the amount of intellectual activity in later life. The report concluded that intellectual activity in later life may be beneficial for both brain structure and function. This cautious conclusion was reached because damage related to dementia probably begins decades before an individual is diagnosed. Environmental stressors, medications, and illnesses occur, but many are reversible and intellectual decline can be diminished. The message is clear, neural plasticity is retained as people age. Older people can learn new skills and their performance can improve.

The ACTIVE trial is the most rigorously conducted trial to date that has assessed intellectual training (Hardy et al., 2015). In this trial, 2832 healthy mid-life to older adults were divided into four groups:

- One received training for memory improvement.
- One received training for reasoning.
- One received training with computerized training in speed of processing.
- One was a control group and received no training

In the training, which emphasized visual perception, individuals were asked to identify objects on a screen quickly. The programme got harder with each correct answer. Participants had ten one-hour training sessions conducted in a classroom setting over five weeks. Some received four additional 'booster' sessions one year after the original training, and four more two years after that. The researchers measured intellectual functioning and competency in daily living changes immediately. These measurements were taken again one, two, three, five, and ten years after the training to see how it had affected the participants performance in daily tasks. In 2015, a study reported that participants assigned to the treatment group improved significantly more in neuropsychological performance than did the control group. Treatment participants showed greater improvements than the control group in:

- Processing speed.
- Short-term memory.
- Working memory.
- Problem solving.
- Fluid reasoning assessments.

Participants in the treatment group also showed greater improvements on self-reported measures of cognitive functioning. This was notable on items related to concentration compared to the control group. This is the first time an intellectual training intervention has been shown to protect against dementia in a large, randomized, controlled trial (Hardy et al., 2015).

Dementia is a loss of brain ability and mind functionality. The bigger and better developed your brain and mind are to start off with, the lower your risk of dementia; just as in the same way the stronger your bones are to start with the lower the risk you will develop osteoporosis. However, it is not just the size of the brain that matters, it is its reserve, its ability to cope with a challenge or an injury or insult. Some people have greater reserve than others and cope better with issues that occur. Generally, brain reserve refers to the brain's ability to sustain any kind of harm or injury, mini strokes for example, and maintain good functional ability despite the harm or injury sustained. There is strong evidence that increased intellectual activity may prevent or delay dementia.

It is important to understand that in assessing the research on intellectual activity there is a need to consider the concepts of brain reserve and intellectual reserve. A larger brain volume may delay onset of dementia despite the presence of damage. Larger brains start with a greater number of neurons and synapses. People with larger brains may have stayed in education longer, but anyone can continue to learn through life. People with more education are likely to have a higher socioeconomic status, meaning that they may be wealthier, have a healthier lifestyle, and have greater access to healthcare. They may have been exposed to fewer toxins at work, and their brains may be protected from small blood vessel disease in the brain.

Intellectual reserve represents brain function, rather than size; this delays or prevents dementia. If you have you ever seen inside telephone junction box when it is being repaired, you may have been amazed that anyone could join up all those brightly coloured wires correctly. The brain is even more complex, with the brain cells, the neurons, not only joining end to end but being organized in networks. People with more education may develop greater complexity and efficiency of neural networks, meaning if damage occurs in the brain, they can compensate by drawing on a greater reserve of routes through the networks. Processes in the brain, such as memory, decision-making, the ability to judge distance or the height of a curb, visual-spatial, and processing speed are related to highly sophisticated networks containing tens of millions of neurons.

The way in which intellectual activity improves brain performance requires more study. With the increased focus on brain research, more researchers are developing sophisticated neuropsychological tests and neuroimaging techniques. These allow for analysis of brain connectivity. The techniques will be used in future research on the importance of increasing intellectual activity at all stages of the human life cycle. This is a huge and fast-growing research field. In 2012, the use of deep brain simulation as a means of helping to improve memory was reported (Suthana et al., 2012).

The more we study the human mind, the greater the scope for helping people retain, regain, and improve their brain power. This will aid them in making calculations, thinking logically and remembering things.

Effects of 'brain games'

Brain games are a billion-dollar industry. They are computer-based intellectually stimulating activities of questionable benefit. The number of people who play video games has steadily increased in past decades. Even small beneficial effects may have other significant public health implications, not always positive. Physical activity, a proven lifestyle factor that improves health, may be reducing because of the sedentary lifestyle associated with video gaming. In 2014, more than 70 prominent neurology and psychology researchers published a consensus statement critical of the brain training industry, citing its 'frequently exaggerated' marketing:

'We object to the claim that brain games offer consumers a scientifically grounded avenue to reduce or reverse cognitive decline when there is no compelling scientific evidence to date that they do,' the statement reads. 'The promise of a magic bullet detracts from the best evidence to date, which is that cognitive health in old age reflects the long-term effects of healthy, engaged lifestyles. In the judgment of the signatories, exaggerated and misleading claims exploit the anxiety of older adults about impending cognitive decline' (Stanford Center on Longevity).

The Luminosity story demonstrates some of the problems that can occur because of over enthusiastic reporting. The Luminosity programme consisted of 40 games purportedly designed to target and train specific areas of the brain. The marketers advertised that playing these games for 10–15 minutes, three or four times a week could help users achieve their 'full potential in every aspect of life'. However, as a result of a Federal Trade Commission decision in early 2016, Luminosity was no longer allowed to make such claims. They could no longer claim that cognitive ability would be improved, and performance increased through use of these games. Nor did they offer protection from physical, age-related, or psychological illnesses that can affect thinking and memory, such as Alzheimer's disease. Companies should only make claims based on high-quality scientific research when it is performed by qualified professionals, independent from the company. This had not taken place, so Luminosity and its representatives could not call their product or a similar one 'clinically proven'.

However, the 'brain games' industry is growing. These 'brain games' do no harm, providing they do not increase the proportion of time sitting as opposed to moving about. If you want to try them, remember that 'brain games' may be no better than other video games. There are also many other things you can do to maintain and improve brain reserve, such as:

- Any form of activity that makes you think, crosswords and sudoku for example.
- Doing activity with other people is even better, playing whist, bridge, or poker is better than playing patience.
- Learning new physical skills helps all aspects of the brain. If you like reading, try painting, if you like music, learn a musical instrument.
- Engagement and argument with other people are both beneficial, the stronger the arguments the better. This is why volunteering is so beneficial. Obviously, a debating club is a good type of organization to join but there are plenty of arguments to be found in everyday life. For example, Alison was a volunteer in a hospital and complained about what she could see was poor clinical care and this led to an enquiry which upset some of the staff but improved care. There is no better example of an activity that will reduce your risk of dementia.

The Harvard Medical School guide to improving Cognitive Fitness, which you can buy online, emphasizes three principles:

- Try something new.
- Challenge yourself; if you have a favourite activity, do something more difficult.
- Vary your cognitive workouts, as you would physical workouts.

Is the need for more social interaction an issue for me?

'Use it or lose it' is a good principle for the brain, mind, and body. Because social interactions require use of more neural networks in your brain, conversations and other activities with friends and family an excellent way for them to help increase your brain reserve. Isolation, whether caused by visual, hearing, or mobility problems, puts people at even higher risk. Everyone should think about ways they can exercise their brain.

Who is there to help?

In yourself

After reading and thinking about your present intellectual activities, write down activities that you would like to pursue that challenge your brain. You might also look for a role model, someone who you feel you can aspire to become because of the challenging brain activities that they are involved in.

In their book *The 100-Year Life* the authors Lynda Gratton and Andrew Scott emphasize the importance of the assets that we acquire while growing up and growing older. Similarly, in the third edition of their bestselling book *Manage Your Mind; The Mental Fitness Guide* (Butler et al., 2018) Tony Hope, Nick Grey, and Gillian Butler give encouragement to becoming more active and involved.

In the community

For many years now, the concept of 'universities for the third age' have been offered in many communities. The idea began in France and the University of the Third Age is now an international movement that aims to educate and stimulate retired members of the community (those in their third 'age' of life). It is commonly referred to as U3A. There is no universally accepted model for U3A, but groups of people in their third age come together to continue their enjoyment of learning in subjects that interest them. An interesting feature of U3A is that there is no distinction between the learners and the teachers. Everyone can take a turn at being both if they wish.

Baby boomers are now staying in the workforce longer, either in full-time or part-time work and the number of new companies started by people aged 60 is increasing all the time. This is another excellent way of exercising your brain daily.

One of the best 'use it or lose it' studies, was conducted by a team in Scotland working in Healthy Ageing in Scotland (HAGIS) (Douglas & Bell, 2019). Their study found no correlation between self-reported use of activities designed to provide intellectual stimulation and reported that the most important thing was to reach a high level of ability in early life. They also recommended to continue with problem solving throughout life. The more difficult the problem, the better. The most difficult challenges in life come not from Sudoku but from other people. Simone De Beauvoir emphasized in her book: *The Coming of Age* (De Beauvoir, 1972) that it is important 'to go on pursuing ends that give our existence a meaning—devotion to individuals, to groups, or to causes—social, political, intellectual, or creative work'.

Get even more active and involved

The benefit from being involved with other people and avoiding isolation is that it keeps the brain healthy and, for many people, prevents depression and feelings of loneliness. Of these three factors, isolation is a simple description of how many people feel who we have met. Depression and loneliness are emotions that influence how well we feel, think, and make decisions.

The brain's resilience and reserve are more likely to be strengthened by meeting more people. Even more so than by simply sitting on your own learning a new skill. The effort of interacting with others calls upon multiple networks in your brain, ensuring that you 'use them and don't lose them'. Evidence is accumulating that meeting and helping people improves cognitive functioning and reduces feelings of loneliness. Imaging studies also show that it reduces the rate of shrinkage of your brain. People who have dementia need more social contact and stimulation than people who do not. Not only should their physical health be optimized but a clear plan is needed to ensure good vision and hearing to keep intellectually engaged and be involved with other people. This can be done face to face and online, and should help people deal with depression, not just accept it as part of ageing.

How does isolation increase the risk of dementia?

Humans are social animals (see Figure 5.4). We engage with our families, work colleagues, and friends, support others and live through the

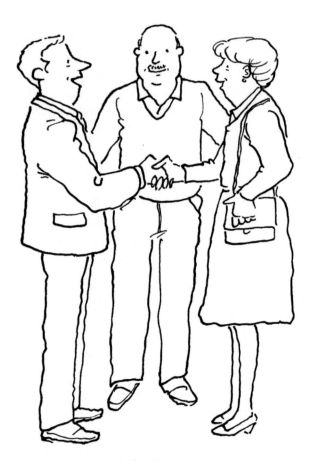

Figure 5.4 Humans are social beings.
Source the Optimal Ageing Programme.

social stresses and strains that this involves. The complexity of social interaction is thought to be the reason for our large forebrain. As humans,
we have done well because of our capacity to manage our social systems
when living in groups and using language in these processes, although
human beings have also done dreadful things to one another in social
groups.

Social and physical factors are connected to loneliness, social isolation, and depression and they contribute to either good or poor cognitive
health, including the amount of cognitive stimulation.

A study of London taxi drivers demonstrated that the brain expands to meet the intellectual demand put on it (Maguire & Woolett, 2011). Similarly, a study of 429,000 former workers in France found that the risk of developing dementia declined with each additional year worked beyond an average retirement age (Dufouil et al., 2013). A 28-year follow-up of the Whitehall II cohort study found a protective effect of social contact against dementia and that more frequent contact confers higher cognitive reserve (Sommerlad et al., 2019). Furthermore, evidence now indicates that individuals lacking social connections are at risk for premature mortality.

What factors improve social functioning?

It is often said that there are two aspects to the mind: emotive, concerned with feeling, and cognitive, concerned with remembering, decision-making, and logical thinking. Cognitive stimulation can be achieved through a variety of activities such as:

- Physical games.
- Childhood reminiscences.
- Current affairs.
- Being creative.
- Using money.
- Number or word games.
- Team quizzes.

In many situations, individuals who are lonely and socially isolated do not have the benefits of cognitive stimulation and in numerous studies cognitive stimulation has been shown to be a cost-effective intervention to improve our thinking abilities. But as we have emphasized in the previous chapter the best type of cognitive stimulation is being with other people even if they are annoying, or perhaps particularly if they are annoying.

Having a safe environment

Loneliness and social isolation cause stress, which can increase your cognitive demand. Stress is caused by living alone when frail and being concerned about internal and external environments. Anything that can be done to help people have a secure dwelling is helpful.

Physical activity

Loneliness and social isolation are associated with having increased feelings of depression and decreased physical activity. Physical activity is important as it improves cognitive health directly. We described earlier in this book that when depression occurs, people often become less physically and mentally active. They can lose interest in continuing with personal hobbies and day-to-day life activities. Physical activity can reduce depression.

Social interactions of good quality

When there are limited interactions with people who provide meaningful exchanges on a regular basis, social interactions may be reduced to only talking to salespeople who knock at the door. Loneliness and social isolation are associated with fewer social interactions. Of course, for an increasing proportion of older people the Internet is providing a means of increasing interaction.

Good sleep

Not having adequate and restful sleep impairs learning at any age and is responsible for an array of other problems. Loneliness and social isolation often interfere with having a good night's sleep. In turn when higher levels of anxiety and depression occur as a result of isolation, sleep can be further affected

Poverty

Millionaires have fewer problems with social isolation than ordinary people. Many of the problems that occur in old age are caused by poverty.

This is of course not an easy problem for an individual to solve or even reduce. But it is important to acknowledge it and to think of ways in which its impact could be reduced (Cadar et al., 2018).

In addition to these reasons for poorer brain health associated with social isolation and loneliness, it may be difficult to determine which comes first. These risk factors are probably the most difficult to give advice about. This is not because it is unclear what actions have beneficial effects but because the people who are at risk are often unable to act.

How strong is the evidence about the benefits of reducing social isolation, loneliness, and depression?

Neuroscience research is continuing to discover the significance of social engagement and its connection with brain shrinkage. Brain shrinkage is part of the normal ageing process. According to some recent studies, the memory centre in the brain maintains its size when engaged in social activities. For example, a controlled trial that lasted 40 weeks, used 120 community-living older adults in Shanghai, China, and randomly assigned each individual to one of the following four groups:

- Tai Chi.
- Walking on their own.
- Social interaction.
- No intervention (control).

Each trial participant had an MRI assessment of their brain size both before and after the intervention period (Mortimer et al., 2012). Each participant also received a battery of neuropsychological tests administered at baseline, 20 weeks, and 40 weeks. Compared to the control group, which received no intervention, significant increases in brain size were seen in the Tai Chi and social intervention groups. The Tai Chi group also improved on the neuropsychological tests. No differences were observed between the group walking on their own and the 'no intervention' groups.

Another controlled trial focused on older adults who had joined the Experience Corps (Carlson et al., 2015). This is a programme that brings retired people into schools to serve as mentors to young children. They work with teachers to help children learn to read in understaffed school libraries. Social engagement is central to participation in the Experience Corps. Participants have a regular routine that is socially and physically engaging. They work in teams with young people and engage in problem solving. This type of activity provides complex socialization that they would not have if they remained at home. After people retire from their regular employment, the Experience Corps provides complexity and novelty in their daily lives. These qualities tend to disappear once people retire. In a research trial, 111 men and women were assigned either to participate in the Experience Corps (58 of 111) or not to participate in the Experience Corps (53 of 111). MRI scans to measure brain size were taken of their brains at enrolment and then again after 12 and 24 months. Participants also received memory tests. Participants were an average of 67.2 years old, predominantly African American, in good health, came from neighbourhoods with low socioeconomic status and had some college education. The control group, those not involved in the Experience Corps, exhibited age-related shrinkage in brain size. Typically, annual rates of brain shrinkage in adults aged over 65 range from 0.8% to 2%. The men who were enrolled in Experience Corps, however, showed a 0.7–1.6% increase in brain size over the course of two years. Though not statistically significant, women appeared to experience small gains, when compared to decline in the control group of 1% over 24 months. At the same time, those with larger increases in the brain size over two years also had the greatest improvements on memory tests. This showed a direct correlation between brain volume and the reversal of a type of cognitive decline associated with increased risk for dementia.

The Shanghai study and Experience Corps studies are intervention studies that showed the importance of social engagement on brain health.

As the contribution of meeting and helping people through increased Brainability research becomes available, more knowledge will become available about specific actions that overcome social isolation, loneliness, and depression.

Is this an issue for me?

Here is an inspiring report of how someone prevented social isolation and reduced the risk that loneliness and depression would contribute to dementia.

Case report

Ed, aged 88, managed to keep focused on the aspects of his life that were important to him. This included caring for his dog Charlie and taking newspapers and his garden produce to the care home staff where his wife Norma lived during the last two years of her life.

As a caring individual, Ed was devoted to visiting Norma daily at the care home. His inner strength and compassion enabled him to accept and deal with watching her deteriorate.

Ed was well liked in his circle of relatives and friends because of his dry sense of humour, his positive beliefs, and his philosophical attitude. He always had a 'can do' approach to issues or problems and this contributed to his ability to be able to live independently in the three years after Norma was not around.

For relatives and friends, Ed was fun to be with because he was always curious. This was particularly evident with his gardening, where he constantly researched new seeds, new seed companies, and new and different approaches to nurturing plants. His garden was the envy of everyone in his neighbourhood and his relatives. He generously donated much of his garden produce to his family and friends.

Ed was never a formal community leader holding a position in some organization, but he participated in local events faithfully. His ability to live alone testified to his thoughtful approach to life. For example, phone calls that were suspicious were detected quickly by him. He dealt with tradespeople around the house and benefited by his ability to communicate and work with them to the satisfaction of all.

Ed is a role model of an older adult who successfully lived his later years independently in his home, guarding against loneliness and social isolation. He was able to achieve an adequate quantity and quality of social connections. He was also able to enhance his sense of purpose and self-esteem, improving his life satisfaction, happiness, and well-being.

What can I do to increase my social activity?

The French philosopher Jean Paul Sartre, said, 'Hell is other people'; while Shakespeare held the view that: 'the mind is its own place and can make a heaven of hell or a hell of heaven.' There you have two ends of the spectrum. The true position is, as usual, somewhere in the middle. Other people are important, but how individuals respond to diminished contact with other people is influenced by their personality. It is also altered by the resources that a person has developed over the years. In their book, *The 100-Year Life*, Lynda Gratton and Andrew Scott (Gratton & Scott, 2016) emphasize that although the word 'assets' is usually used to mean financial assets, people acquire other assets as they grow older. They can continue to learn new skills or productive assets, to use their useful language, throughout life. One of the key messages of their book is that we are moving from a world in which there are three phases of life, education, work, and retirement. Within the new approach many people will change their occupation several times, losing old skills and learning new skills in midlife or after. Another type of 'asset' they write about is the transformational 'asset' which they define as the ability to cope with change and challenges. Some people will cope better with the onset of deafness or isolation than others, due to the skills they have acquired. It is important to emphasize that:

- Even people who have these skills may give up because they wrongly believe that 'nothing can be done' when the term dementia is mentioned. The fact is, people who do have dementia are even more in need of social contact and stimulation than people who do not.
- Everyone who develops dementia needs to optimize their physical health. Clear plans must also be made to ensure that their vision and hearing are kept as good as possible.

Friends and family

People do not always choose to become isolated. It can be forced upon them by disabling health problems or a lack of money. The person who has plenty of money is rarely isolated. This could be because they may be more attractive to a certain type of visitor, but more likely because they have the resources to get extra help if they need it. They also have the resources to travel in comfort if they can no longer drive or use public transport.

People do not choose to become depressed or lonely. These moods develop due to several factors. Some are obvious and understandable, death of a partner for example. They can also come out of the blue; the relationship between loneliness and depression is complex. What is clear is that isolation greatly increases the risk of both. A major cause of isolation is population mobility. Spring Chicken is a company that has been set up specifically to help people trying to support a parent or parents hundreds of miles away.

In the community

Community engagement studies report that depression is reduced when people feel valued and appreciated for their formal volunteering roles (Byers & Yaffe, 2011). Several opportunities are available which individuals can use to reduce feelings of depression. However, even these require the motivation to start the programme.

Meeting and helping people can include activities of neighbourliness, such as informally helping with shopping or visiting an old person who has no relatives in a care home. There are also formal activities, such as volunteering for nature conservation group, or civic roles, such as becoming a school trustee (see Figure 5.5). Making contributions to community life does not guarantee that this will protect against social isolation and frailty later in life. According to a review by the Centre for Ageing Better entitled: *The Benefits of Making a Contribution to Your Community in Later Life* (Jones et al., 2016), studies have shown that less well connected, healthy, or wealthy people benefit more by becoming

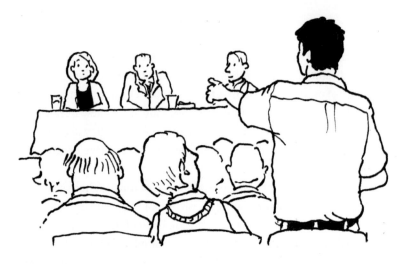

Figure 5.5 Emotional health and thinking ability benefits from meeting, helping, and arguing with people.
Source the Optimal Ageing Programme.

engaged in the community. This is compared to those who are already connected, healthy, and wealthy.

In the health service

For some lonely, isolated, or depressed people the health service is their main opportunity to be in meaningful contact with other human beings. Further, health service providers can provide information about ways to overcome loneliness, feelings of isolation, and depression. They do this through interventions, such as psychotherapy, meditation, self-help groups, and other non-pharmacological interventions. These are available in the community and provide help for lonely, isolated, or depressed people. This support can also include cognitive behavioural therapy (CBT) delivered by a psychologist. Anti-depressant drugs have a part to play, but should only be prescribed after all the other interventions described here have been tried and continued, even after medication has been prescribed. If a person has thoughts of suicide or speaks about suicide, they should see their doctor as soon as possible.

Keep your hearing and vision sharp

New findings about neurologic mechanisms from brain imaging studies help explain how uncorrected deficits in vision and hearing can lead to cognitive decline. People who cannot see or hear well often become socially isolated and deprived of stimuli that keep the brain cognitively engaged.

Vision is associated with a good functioning brain and poor vision leads to cognitive decline. As we age, some visual problems occur that can be corrected with glasses, but diseases of the eye are more frequent in older adults and should be identified and treated by eye specialists. By sustaining one's hearing and improving vision it is possible to avoid or at least delay the consequences of hearing and vision loss that include communication difficulties, social isolation, depression, an increased risk of falls, decline in physical functioning, dementia, and a decreased quality of life. Vision and hearing can be sustained through actions taken by the individual, their family and friends, the community, and health practitioners.

What is good-quality vision and hearing?

Some people age without ever experiencing changes in their vision, but there are some vision changes that are common with the natural ageing of the eye. These can include: difficulty seeing objects clearly, even close up; a decline in colour sensitivity, such as being able to distinguish colours such as blue from black; and the need for more light when reading. These changes can often be corrected with a new prescription for glasses or improved lighting. However, older adults should know the difference between changes that are normal and those that are not.

The most common eye diseases and conditions that affect older adults include age-related macular degeneration (AMD), cataract, diabetic retinopathy, glaucoma, and dry eye.

Deafness is a much worse misfortune than loss of vision. Helen Keller famously noted in a 1910 letter to Dr James Love: 'The problems of deafness are deeper and more complex, if not more important, than those of blindness. For it means the loss of the most vital stimulus—the sound of the voice that brings language, sets thoughts astir and keeps us in the intellectual company of man' (Keller & Love, 1933). She was pointing out that decreased quality of life from loss of hearing involves communication difficulties, social isolation, and depression.

Hearing loss includes difficulty understanding speech, especially if the speech is distorted or embedded in noise, problems related to localizing sound, being able to hear with both ears, and increased sensitivity to loudness. Presbycusis, or normal age-related hearing loss, worsens slowly, affects both ears, but usually only results in difficulty hearing high-pitched sounds. Hearing loss is due to three causes:

- Degeneration of the cochlea or inner ear, called peripheral hearing loss.
- Central hearing loss due to brain disease, occurring much less frequently.
- Conductive hearing loss in the middle and outer ear, which is the most common type of hearing loss. Conductive hearing loss in older adults can occur due to extreme wax build-up.

Only 2% of the older population has central hearing loss according to the Lancet Commission on Dementia Prevention and Care (Livingston et al., 2017). In contrast, peripheral hearing loss in the older population is much more common at 28%, 43%, and 58%, depending on the specific study.

According to the Lancet Commission on Dementia Prevention and Care, hearing loss is grouped with the other midlife risks of dementia, namely hypertension and obesity (Livingston et al., 2017). The study found that hearing loss increased the risk of developing dementia more than several of the other individual risks. These included: the level of childhood education, exercise, maintaining social engagement, reducing or stopping smoking, management of hearing loss, depression, and diabetes.

How strong is the evidence that good-quality vision and hearing reduces the risk of dementia?

University of Michigan researchers Mary Rogers and Kenneth Langa (2010) reported that older people with poor vision had a 63% greater risk of developing dementia over a period of eight and a half years. Those with poor vision who did not visit an ophthalmologist were five times more likely to experience cognitive decline and nine times more likely to develop dementia.

Eye diseases may have no early symptoms. Evidence suggests that everyone aged over fifty should have regular comprehensive dilated eye examinations. Early detection, treatment, and follow-up care are important to preventing vision loss and blindness.

In a study of older adults Dr Frank Lin and his colleagues at Johns Hopkins University, found that those who had hearing loss were 24% more likely to experience cognitive decline within six years. Their cognitive abilities declined up to 40% faster than others with normal hearing (Lin et al., 2013). They had greater problems with brain functions, such as reasoning and memory, developing them an average of three years earlier. The more severe their hearing loss at the start of the study, the greater their cognitive loss over time. These findings occurred while controlling for diseases like diabetes and high blood pressure.

In a more recent study of 154,414 adults aged 50 and above, who had health insurance claims, Dr Lin and his colleagues found that untreated hearing loss increased the risk of developing dementia by 50%. Depression also increased by 40% in five years when compared to those without hearing loss. In 2019, as part of another study (Reed et al., 2019), Dr Lin and his colleagues reported that untreated hearing loss increases healthcare cost and utilization. This conclusion was based on data from a healthcare claims database. Persons with untreated hearing loss experienced more inpatient stays and were at greater risk for 30-day hospital readmission at ten years later. Similar trends were observed at two and five-year time points.

How hearing and vision loss cause cognitive impairment and dementia

Functional magnetic resonance imaging (MRI) studies (more detailed than conventional MRI), are revealing that people with even mild hearing loss use more of their frontal cortex when trying to understand speech. This means that the part of the brain needed for thinking and decision-making is overworked. Even with mild hearing loss, the hearing areas of the brain become weaker. What happens next is that some areas of the brain, such as the frontal cortex, which are necessary for higher level thinking, compensate for the weaker areas. These areas step in and essentially take over for hearing, leaving them unavailable to enable the individual to do well with memory, thinking, and decision-making.

The link between good vision and hearing and dementia could be due to three processes:

- 'Cognitive load', when you can see or hear well. The brain is receiving clear signals and is not forced to work harder in order to derive meaning from the message.
- Individuals who continue to become socially engaged prevent diminished cognitive stimulation and cognitive loss. People with vision and hearing problems are more likely to become isolated.
- Hearing and seeing well helps avoid brain shrinkage mostly of the hearing portion of the brain, which also is involved in functions like memory, learning and thinking.

In addition, vision and hearing loss may result from changes to a vulnerable brain, for example a brain not fully operational because of blood vessel disease.

Oxford University epidemiologists, Richard Doll and Richard Peto, proposed a model in cancer research that suggested rapid changes in the occurrence of a health problem in a population over time. Increases or decreases were strong indicators that the health problem was preventable. They pointed out that genetic changes accrue slowly and affect health over long periods of time. However, their model identifies that environmental or behavioural factors can change suddenly. The good news, based on this principle, is that the Epidemiology of Hearing Loss

Study and the Beaver Dam Offspring Study found that older adults are retaining good hearing longer than previous generations. This indicates that changes in the environment (e.g. less noise at work) and behaviours (such as reduced smoking prevalence) may account for this change.

Finally, hearing can be improved with assistive listening devices, including telephone or mobile phone amplifying devices, smart phone or tablet apps, and closed-circuit systems (induction coil loops). Closed-circuit systems are being used in places of worship, theatres, and auditoriums. The quality of the evidence is complicated, especially when determining the effectiveness of hearing aids, assistive listening devices, and surgically placed amplification devices (such as middle ear implants and cochlear implants). The studies are complicated due to the fact that with more severe degrees of hearing loss, conventional hearing aids increase auditory awareness without substantially improving speech discrimination or communicative ability. The amount of benefit from hearing aids also depends on the type of hearing aid used, hours worn per day, number of years used. The characteristics of participants choosing to use hearing aids also influence this, in addition to the use of other communicative strategies and adequacy of rehabilitation.

Randomized trials to determine whether hearing aids can prevent or delay dementia's onset are also complicated. Only a minority of people with hearing loss are either diagnosed or treated, and when prescribed, many people do not use their hearing aids. Thus, a randomized trial could not simply assign one group to use a hearing aid. However, trials may be feasible if linked to a programme entitled Hearing Equality through Accessible Research and Solutions (HEARS). HEARS uses visual materials and training for the participant and a family member to increase hearing aid use in cognitively healthy older adults. Evaluations have found that the programme increases hearing aid use.

As with hearing aids, it is not known whether cochlear implants can prevent or delay dementia's onset. Recent reviews found only three studies, none of which reported positive neurocognitive outcomes following cochlear implantation surgery in adults aged over 65 years. Nor did they include control groups without cochlear implants. A recent population study from France reported improvements in hearing loss and in speech recognition abilities after cochlear implantation. Studies with comparison groups are needed as surgical procedures in cochlear implantation have advanced in recent years. These advancements have made stimulator-receivers less bulky, surgical tools for cochlear insertions more refined, and operative magnification and lighting have improved. These factors all allow for smaller incisions and dramatically shortened operative times when compared to earlier generations of technology.

Trials of cochlea implants are complicated further by the fact that few people have them. A recent review reported that only 5–10% of adult cochlear implant candidates in the USA have received cochlear implants. This is despite eligible coverage by Medicare for persons aged 65 and over and many insurance carriers currently pay for the procedure. Approximately 50,000 cochlear implant surgeries are performed per year worldwide based on manufacturer revenue estimates; about 20,000–25,000 of these are used in adults. The most rapidly growing segment receiving cochlear implants are those aged over 65, but the average delay between onset of hearing loss to receiving a cochlear implant in adults is estimated to be ten years.

In order to invest in future good quality vision and hearing, prevention should start in midlife. Begin with exercise, maintaining social engagements, and reducing or stopping smoking. Managing depression, diabetes, hypertension, and obesity will also help, in addition to acting on poor-quality hearing.

What you can do to protect your vision

According to a review of the evidence by the Canadian National Institution for the Blind Foundation, lifetime investing in good vision will be maintained and eye diseases avoided by adopting the following strategies:

Prevention strategy reproduced with the permission of the Canadian National Institute for the Blind—the CNIB Foundation (2021)

- Quitting smoking. Through adopting this strategy, you will become three to four times less likely to develop age-related macular degeneration since smoking is a major risk factor for this disease (even reducing the number of cigarettes smoked per day will help). Smoking and a family history of age-related macular degeneration is a particularly potent risk combination. It will reduce the risk of developing diabetic retinopathy if you have diabetes, and it will also be easier to control your blood pressure and sugar levels. You will also be less likely to develop cataracts.

- Improving your diet and maintaining a healthy weight. This reduces the risk of developing age-related macular degeneration. You should avoid foods high in unsaturated fats and those that are highly processed or refined and increase your intake of whole grains, foods high in omega-3s, fresh fruit, and dark green leafy vegetables. By extension this lowers your risk of diabetes, and diabetic retinopathy.
- Reducing sunlight exposure. This protects the eye's retina and reduce chances of developing age-related macular degeneration and cataracts. When out in the sun, wear sunglasses with 100% UV protection, even in winter.
- Preventing diabetes reduces your risk of many kinds of vision loss. Most people with diabetes are at a high risk of developing diabetic retinopathy and other vision problems.
- Managing diabetes (if you already have it), significantly lowers your risk of developing diabetic retinopathy. It's particularly crucial if you have type 1 diabetes to control your blood pressure, sugar, and lipid (fat) levels.
- Drinking in moderation will reduce the risk of developing cataracts, since heavy drinking of alcoholic beverages is a known risk factor.
- Taking steps to avoid eye injuries. Protect yourself from cataracts. Injuries may include a hard blow, puncture, cut, intense heat, or a chemical burn. Wear eye protection when doing sports, home repairs, or other activities that could put your eyes at risk. You should also work in a well-ventilated area if you are using chemicals.
- Getting regular eye exams. Become much more likely to catch age-related macular degeneration, glaucoma, and diabetic retinopathy in the early stages, where they often have no noticeable symptoms. If you catch them early, treatment options are better, and you have a better chance to save much more of your vision.

Lifetime investing in good hearing can be achieved by turning down the volume. Consider setting volume control limits on all devices and do not always have the music on to give the ears time to recover. Wearing hearing protection when using power tools or travelling can also help. Studies have shown that frequent exposure to subways and train noises can lead to permanent hearing loss. You can also learn how to play a musical instrument or join a choir. Recent studies show that playing a musical instrument through adulthood helps to maintain listening skills. These allow us to understand what a person is saying in noisy environments, such as in a coffee shop or restaurant.

If your hearing quality has decreased, you can work on becoming a more effective communicator. Learn to take charge of your communication assertively but not aggressively. There are many ways to be assertive, for example you can ask people to get your attention before speaking to you, suggest that they face you, or ask them not to shout. Another way to be assertive is to learn to use strategies for handling communication breakdowns. You must know when to ask for a 'rephrase' instead of a 'repeat', and how to apply a clarification strategy. Put simply, learn how to ask questions.

Is visual loss an issue for me?

You can assess the quality of your vision if you have difficulty seeing objects clearly, a decline in sensitivity, such as not being able to distinguish colours, or needing more light in order to see.

Is hearing loss an issue for me?

If any of the following statements apply to you, then you may have difficulty hearing and should be seeking help from a health practitioner:

- You sometimes feel embarrassed when you meet new people because you struggle to hear.
- You feel frustrated when talking to members of your family because you have difficulty hearing them.

- You have difficulty hearing when someone speaks in a whisper.
- You feel restricted or limited by a hearing problem.
- You have difficulty hearing when visiting friends, relatives, or neighbours.
- A hearing problem causes you to attend faith organization services less often than you would like.
- Hearing problems cause you to argue with family members.
- You have trouble hearing the TV or radio at levels that are loud enough for others.
- You feel that any difficulty with your hearing limits your personal or social life.
- You have trouble hearing family or friends when you are together in a restaurant. (Ventry & Weinstein, 1982)

Who can support me?

In friends and family

You and your family can work together to make vision and hearing easier. You can tell your friends and family about your vision or hearing loss; they need to know that these are hard for you. The more you tell the people you spend time with, the more they can help you. If you have poor vision, ask your friends and family to ensure good lighting in the places where you meet. If you have a poor hearing, ask your friends and family to face you when they talk to you so that you can see their faces. If you watch their faces move and see their expressions, it may help you to understand them better. You can also ask people to speak more loudly, but not shout. They do not have to talk slowly, just more clearly. Turning off the TV or radio when you are not actively listening to them can also help. Be aware of noise around you that can make hearing more difficult. When you go to a restaurant, do not sit near the kitchen or near a band playing music, as background noise makes it hard to hear people talk. Working together to see or hear better may be tough on everyone for a while and will take time for you to get used to. Be patient and continue to work together. Hearing and seeing better are worth the effort.

In the community

In addition to health charities who provide services to those with hearing and vision impairments, you might also consider help from your peers. Seeking out others in the community who share in visual and hearing difficulties will enable them to relate and empathize with you better than others might. Depending on the context of your poor-quality vision or hearing dilemma, the characteristics of the peer that may be most helpful are someone your age, gender, place of residence, or culture. The key issue is that the peer is your equal.

In the health service

After you have engaged in trying to resolve your poor-quality vision or hearing, received help from friends and family, and community assistance, but feel as though nothing has worked, it might be time to consult a professional. For hearing problems an audiologist is the first person to consult. Their first step will be to exclude wax as the cause of the problem. If this is not the cause of the hearing impairment, they will start the process of assessing the benefit that a hearing aid and support service could offer. It is important not to see the hearing aid as simply a piece of technology. It takes time to adjust to the hearing aid and to learn how to use it. It is the personal service that is as important as the actual aid. The audiologist can also advise on the need for specialist advice or referral to an ear, nose, and throat department because only they can assess the need for a cochlear implant. Audiologists are educators and can teach you ways to improve communication in difficult listening situations, as in the situations previously listed in this chapter.

For visual problems, see an optometrist. For sudden loss of vision in one or both eyes, go straight to the eye hospital emergency department. People aged over 50 should be seeing an optometrist regularly and the common problems such as cataracts, age-related macular degeneration (AMD), and glaucoma will be detected at these visits. If you have diabetes type 1 or 2, you will be receiving separate invitations for screening to detect retinopathy. If the optometrist thinks specialist advice and assessment is necessary, they will make the necessary arrangements.

Watch this space: Developments for which there is not yet evidence of effectiveness

Physical activity is good for the brain both directly and indirectly. This is through keeping your arteries open and healthy. The evidence about the benefits of mental and social activity is more difficult to generate because the research is more difficult to organize, but it, too, is getting stronger.

The previous comments made about Lumosity should not put you off brain exercise.

As outlined at the beginning of this book, dementia becomes problematic when four key functions are affected:

- Looking after your financial affairs.
- Self-care and maintaining personal hygiene.
- Cleaning and maintaining a living space.
- Driving.

Fortunately, there is evidence of the benefits from computer-based training on the ability to reason logically and the speed of processing information that can all contribute to these four functions. Using a measurement called useful field of vision (UFOV), it has been shown that a person can be stimulated to act quickly when images appear at the edge of what they can see flashing up on the screen. This can improve the speed with which you see and react to a potential threat, such as a car appearing at speed from a side street. The improvement in speed of reaction is so great that some insurers in the USA have started to ask their clients over a certain age to undertake this form of training.

The evaluation of maintaining or increasing social activity is where the most progress is likely to be seen, with increasing expectation that people who are living longer will stay active longer, doing socially useful voluntary work if not in employment or starting a new business. Even housebound older people can contribute. These contributions can be made through gathering data in research projects that require human rather than artificial intelligence, for example projects such as those organized by Zooniverse. The key is to stay engaged and new technology includes virtual reality (VR).

Virtual Reality

Imagine someone who is 84 and housebound. The priority should be to help them get out more often. However, the Internet offers opportunities to supplement face-to-face contact. These advancements make it possible to access knowledge and, with a combination of Alexa Skill software (from Amazon Web Services) or Zoom (on an iPhone) and virtual reality, they could:

- Cycle with Zwift every morning as part of a VR group, cycling from Land's End to John O'Groats. Their group could raise money to combat climate change or fund cancer research, or compete with other groups of older people. More importantly they would be in a group with a purpose.
- Join a book club listening to Inspector Morse on Audible and join a discussion group about writing detective fiction.

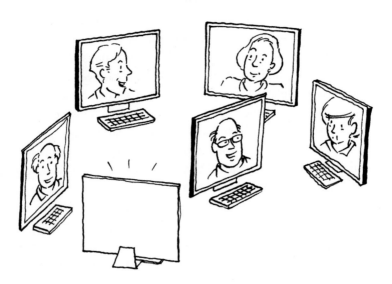

Figure 5.6 Social engagement can occur through use of your computer to connect with others.
Source the Optimal Ageing Programme.

- Do a virtual tour of Oxford's Natural History Museum, which they would have to do standing up, using a treadmill to walk and climb stairs when that was required.
- Use their Wizdish treadmill and the virtual walk app to continue their guided walk along the Great Wall of China or raise funds for a charity by a sponsored walk along the Thames Path or the West Highland Way.
- Join a concert party in the evening for music and a discussion before starting their pre-sleep ritual.

The key appears to be engagement, real always in preference to virtual (see Box 5.1). However, the stimulation of being able to experience things through the Internet with other people should not be underestimated (see Figure 5.6).

Of the three means of improving Brainability and reducing the risk of dementia this is the one that is most complex, while at the same time

---

Box 5.1   Free high-quality systematic reviews of the evidence

- Yates, L.A., Ziser, S., Spector, A., & Orrell, M. (2016). Cognitive leisure activities and future risk of cognitive impairment and dementia: systematic review and meta-analysis. *International Psychogeriatrics*, 28(11), 1791–1806. doi: https://doi.org/10.1017/S1041610216001137.
- Global Council on Brain Health (2017). *The Brain and Social Connectedness: GCBH Recommendations on Social Engagement and Brain Health 2017.* Available at www.GlobalCouncilOnBrainHealth.org
- Holt-Lunstad, J., Smith, T.B., Baker, M., Harris, T., & Stephenson, D. (2015). Loneliness and social isolation as risk factors for mortality: A meta-analytic review. *Perspectives on Psychological Science*, 10(2), 227–237.
- Holt-Lunstad, J., Smith, T.B., & Layton, J.B. (2010). Social Relationships and Mortality Risk: A Meta-analytic Review. *PLoS Med* 7(7), e1000316. https://doi.org/10.1371/journal.pmed.

Continued

Box 5.1 *Continued*

- Sommerlad, et al. (2019). Association of social contact with dementia and cognition: 28-year follow-up of the Whitehall II cohort study. *PLOS Medicine,* https://doi.org/10.1371/journal.pmed.1002862.
- Da Silva, J., et al. (2013). Affective disorders and risk of developing dementia: Systematic review. *British Journal of Psychiatry,* 202(3), 177–86. doi: 10.1192/bjp.bp.111.101931.
- Dawes, P., et al. (2019). Interventions for hearing and vision impairment to improve outcomes for people with dementia: a scoping review. *International Psychogeriatrics,* 31(2), 203–221. doi: 10.1017/S1041610218000728. Epub 24 Sept. 2018.

offering the easiest means of implementation. The scientific literature is also complex and for this reason we include several references which provide not only knowledge but also insight into the way scientists are thinking about isolation, loneliness, and their impact on brain function and dementia.

References

Butler, G., Grey, N., & Hope, T. (2018). *Manage Your Mind.* Oxford: Oxford University Press.

Byers, A.L. & Yaffe, K. (2011). Depression and risk of developing dementia. *Nature Reviews Neurology,* 6, 323–331.

Carlson, M.C., Kuo, J.H., Chuang, Y., Varma, V., Harris, G. (2015). Impact of the Baltimore Experience Corps Trial on cortical and hippocampal volumes. *Alzheimer's & Dementia,* 11, 1340–1348.

Cadar D, et al. (2018). Individual and area-based socioeconomic factors associated with dementia incidence in England evidence from a 12-year follow-up in the English Longitudinal Study of Ageing. *Journal of American Medical Association of Psychiatry,* 75, 723–732.

CNIB Foundation. (2021). https://www.cnib.ca/en/sight-loss-info/your-eyes/eye-health?region=on

De Beauvoir, S. (1972). *The Coming of Age.* André Deutsch Ltd and George Weidenfeld and Nicolson Ltd, London.

Douglas, E. & Bell, D. (2019). The relationship between loneliness, social isolation and health service usage in an older population: an example of administrative data linkage using Healthy Ageing In Scotland (HAGIS) and NHS records. *International Journal of Population Data Science,* 4(3).

Dufouil, C., Pereira, E., Chene, G., Gilmour, M.M., Saubusse, E., et al. (2014). Older age at retirement is associated with decreased risk of dementia: Analysis of a health care insurance database of self-employed workers. *European Journal of Epidemiology*, 29(5), 353–361.

Gratton, L. & Scott, A. (2016). *The 100-Year Life. Living and Working in an Age of Longevity*. Bloomsbury, London.

Hardy, J.L., Nelson, R.A., Thomason, M.A., Sternberg, D.A., Katovich, K., Farzin, F. (2015). Enhancing cognitive abilities with comprehensive training: large, online, randomized, active-controlled trial. *PLoS ONE*, 9, e0134467.

Jones, D.,Young, A., Reeder, N. (2016). *The Benefits of Making a Contribution to Your Society in Later Life*. The Centre for Ageing Better, London.

Keller, H. & Love, J.K. (1933). *Helen Keller in Scotland*. Methuen, London.

Lin, F., Yaffe, K., Xia, J., Xue, Q., Harris, T.B., Purchase-Zelner, E. (2013). Hearing loss and cognitive decline in older adults. *Journal of American Medical Association* 173(4), 293–299.

Livingston, G., Sommerlad, A., Orgeta, V., Costa Freda, S.G., Huntley, J., Ames, D., et al. (2017). The Lancet Commission on 'Dementia prevention, intervention, and care'. *Lancet*, 390, 2673–2734.

Maguire, E.A. & Woolett, K. (2011). Acquiring 'the knowledge' of London's layout drives structural brain changes. *Current Biology*, 21, 2109–2114.

Mortimer, J.A., Ding, D., Borenstein, A.R., DeCarli, C., Guo, Q., Zhao, Q. (2012). Changes in brain volume and cognition in a randomized trial of exercise and so-cial interaction in a community-based sample of non-demented Chinese elders. *Journal of Alzheimer's Disease*, 4, 757–766.

Prince, M., Albanese, E., Guerchet, M., Prina, M. (2014). *Dementia and Risk Reduction: An Analysis of Protective and Modifiable Factors*. Alzheimer's Disease International, London.

Reed, N.S., Altan, A., Deal, J.A., et al. (2019). Trends in Health Care Costs and Utilization Associated With Untreated Hearing Loss Over 10 Years. *JAMA Otolaryngol Head Neck Surg*, 145(1), 27–34. doi:10.1001/jamaoto.2018.2875

Rogers, M. & Langa, K. (2010). Untreated poor vision: A contributing factor to late-life dementia. *American Journal of Epidemiology*, 6, 728–735.

Stanford Center on Longevity (2014). A Consensus on the Brain Training Industry from the Scientific Community. Stanford University. Available at: http://longevity3.stanford.edu/blog/2014/10/15/the-consensus-on-the-brain-training-industry-from-the-scientific-community-2/

Suthana, N., Haneef, Z., Stern, J., Mukamel, R., Behnke, E., Knowlton, B. (2012). Memory enhancement and deep-brain stimulation of the entorhinal area. *New England Journal of Medicine*, 6, 502–510.

Ventry, I. & Weinstein, B. (1982). The Hearing Handicap Inventory for the elderly. *Ear Hearing*, 3, 128–134.

6

The Future of Brainability

In her book published in 2019 Camilla Cavendish analyses what is happening, and what needs to happen, as populations age. The book is cleverly called *Extra Time* (Cavendish, 2019), the period of a football (soccer) match in which the game could go either way, and describes ten lessons for us to learn if we want to stand a better chance of winning, that is increase our healthspan and reduce our risk of dementia. Cavendish also reviews the evidence about the importance of having a sense of purpose, building on the key Japanese concept of Ikigai (translated as life purpose). This presents a challenging but encouraging view of what is going on and what needs to be done to help people live better longer. Here are her ten insights:

- Demography tips the balance of power.
- The stages of life are changing.
- If exercise and diet was a pill, we'd all be taking it.
- Don't give up the day job.
- Old brains can learn new tricks—and they must to keep in shape.
- Immortality isn't here yet, but anti-ageing drugs are on the way.
- Everyone needs a neighbourhood.
- Robots care for you—humans care about you.
- Purpose is vital.
- We need a new social contract.

In this book we have focused on you, the reader, but the individual must live in society. It is society that creates the environment, both social and physical, which influences many of the decisions that individuals make. Perhaps the strongest message is the influence of others. Currently the population is top-heavy, with the number of people aged over 65

Increase your Brainability—and Reduce your Risk of Dementia. Charles Alessi, Larry W. Chambers, and Muir Gray, Oxford University Press. © Oxford University Press 2021. DOI: 10.1093/oso/9780198860341.003.0006

outnumbering the number of people aged five or under for the first time since records began.

As people live longer, the stages of life change and there are no longer the three classic phases of education, work, and retirement. We are experiencing what Lynda Gratton and Andrew Scott called, a 'multi-phase life' (Gratton & Scott, 2016). This has led to civil disturbance in France due to the pension age being raised; however, some are delaying their pension by declining retirement. Some are even starting a new career. The Council of the Royal College of Surgeons discussed the paradox of the National Health Service having a shortage of surgeons while at the same time requiring all surgeons to retire at 65. There is no evidence that all surgeons lose manual dexterity at that age. The pension age was determined and remains determined by actuaries not by physical or mental ability.

Development in our knowledge of basic biological changes and their genetic origins is producing new tests that may be useful. It is now thought that whatever our genetic predisposition, there is much we can do to reduce our risk of developing dementia. The emergence of biomarkers is a new area of science. These reflect our risks and are affected by a whole series of factors. Japan, because of a super-ageing society, is particularly interested in ageing; some municipalities have developed scores for their citizens. Kanagawa prefecture, part of greater Tokyo, has developed a new scale called the Me-Byo index which measures how active in risk reduction a citizen has been. This encourages citizens to be more actively engaged in their health by awarding them vouchers for improvements. Methods for detecting slight changes in cognition and early signs of dementia are also an area of research in both Japan and Australia. Both countries have been experimenting with methods of detecting small changes using voice recordings from citizens over the phone. Thus, there is much we can and should do to better manage our risks, but the principal development is the recognition that knowledge is the elixir of life.

Knowledge is increasing, not only about genes and chemicals, but also by applying what we know already about how we can live longer and better. The number and range of books and other sources of knowledge is increasing all the time. These are books about well-being in general, not just about dementia, but the same principles and actions that reduce the risk of one condition like dementia reduce the risk of physical frailty and dependency, and vice versa. In addition to the books in the 'Sod It' series such as *Sod70!* by Muir Gray (2015), look at *When We're 64* by Louise Ansari (2019), and *How to Age Joyfully* by Maggy Piggot (2019), which has eight simple rules:

- Move.
- Eat right.
- Have a purpose.
- Connect.
- Grow.
- Be grateful.
- Give.
- Be positive.

In the Scientific American eBook, *The New Science of Healthy Aging* (Bennett, 2019), David Bennett highlights the different outcome for two women Marge and Mary, who had 'mild tissue loss and enough damage to meet the pathological criteria for Alzheimer's. [Mary] actually had less beta-amyloid and fewer tangles than Marge did. Despite having less Alzheimer's pathology than Marge, Mary suffered from a progressive loss of cognition, resulting in an inability to care for herself by the time of her death.' Whereas Marge continued to be involved, helping others as well as having a full life. This was not just due to a decision that she made at the age of 60. It reflected the big differences in the social and educational background of the two women, leading David Bennet to draw up his list of 'ten things you can do to reduce the risk of losing cognition and developing Alzheimer's dementia:

1. Pick your parents well! Make sure you get good genes, a good education, a second language, and music lessons. Avoid emotional neglect.
2. Engage in regular cognitive and physical activity.
3. Strengthen and maintain social ties.
4. Get out and explore new things.
5. Chillax and be happy.
6. Avoid people who are downers, especially close family members!
7. Be conscientious and diligent.

8. Spend time engaged in activities that are meaningful and goal-directed.
9. Be heart-healthy: what's good for the heart is good for the brain.
10. Eat a MIND diet, with fresh fruit and vegetables and fish.
11. (For fans of This Is Spinal Tap, our list goes to 11.) Be lucky!'

All points except 1 and 11 are relevant for people of any age and it is important to remember that the cover of the Lancet containing their 2020 Dementia Commission Report had only the statement "It is never too early and never too late in the life course for dementia prevention" and in that year the issue of dementia caused by repeated sporting concussion hit not the front page of every newspaper but the back page, the sports page. It has long been recognized that some boxers became 'punch drunk' but the high incidence of early onset dementia in players of American football, soccer and rugby became a major news story in 2020. In rugby the campaign to minimize contact in school rugby had been started by a parent, who was also a public health doctor, Alysson Pollock who published a book titled Tackling Rugby and sub titled, what every parent should know. In 2020, the rugby authorities took steps to miniise contact and to ensure that if a player was concussed they should leave the field and take sufficient time to recover before they next played. In football the death from dementia of some of the members of England's 1966 world cup winning team raised the issue and although the modern ball is much lighter in wet weather that footballs in times past. The authorities recognized that action had to be taken, for example, banning heading in training or by schoolchildren.

As individuals and as a society we can live longer and better; this point is emphasized in the book by Anna Dixon (Director of the Centre of Ageing Better) entitled The Age of Ageing Better (2020) which emphasizes the need to see ageing as a social and political issue as well as a personal issue. All policymakers and politicians should read this Manifesto for Our Future, the subtitle of the book.

The evidence for the preventability of dementia gets stronger and the report of the Lancet Commission on Dementia first published in 2017 strengthened its recommendations in 2020, adding to the list of risk factors heavy drinking, traumatic brain injury, including sports trauma, and air pollution (Lancet, 2020).

How will it affect me?

We live in a world where change is ever present, and the pace of change is increasing exponentially. One hundred years after Richard Arkwright invented the spinning jenny in 1769, the industrial landscape had totally transformed towns and cities. Compare this with the time it has taken for the digital revolution to reach its present frenetic pace. The first mobile call was made in 1973, the agreement on common protocols between computers which led to the Internet was reached in 1983. Now, most of us travel with portable computers in our pocket. The focus is now on robotics, artificial intelligence, and machine learning, with a pace of change that continues to surprise, alarm, and delight in equal measure. We live in a world where machines not only understand language but are starting to infer intent behind the spoken word and driverless cars are predicted to be just around the corner. This digital revolution is leading us all to question the way we do things, and the nature and relevance of many of our national health institutions. What is clear is that we are at the start of a journey which will take us to places we cannot even start to imagine. However, digital developments offer many simpler opportunities than artificial intelligence (AI). For example, the Belgian company Memoride has introduced a virtual reality cycling experience which allows people who cannot get back on the road to cycle down memory lane or along new roads. Even more exciting is the plan to use this technology to allow people to cycle in groups, and for those groups to have a social purpose such as raising money to help children and young people to take action to improve the environment. There is also the proposal for these groups to be competitive, with older people in one home or one town competing with other similar groups to see who can raise the most money for these good causes. This will, however, require action to increase the numbers and proportion of older people who are online and the Covid 19 pandemic has given an important stimulus to the need to do this, and an increased recognition by older people of the need to be online. The impact of decreased activity and increased isolation on mental and physical health during lockdown was recognized by Prime Minister Boris Johnson, when he launched the lockdown policy and will increase the risk of dementia and the need for action to reduce digital exclusion. New technology will make an increasingly important contribution. The Echo

Show and Facebook's portal allow engagement without the need to type or even see and the new Wizdish treadmill which has no moving parts, thus making it very safe, but which has full virtual reality capacity allows people, including people with dementia, living on their own, or in a care home, to walk in wonderful places, with family and friends who may be hundreds or thousands of miles away.

You are likely wondering how this will affect you trying to manage your risk of developing dementia or what you should do about it. The best way to tackle this is to look at the ways we now manage our health and think of how this will look in the future. Also, try to think in terms of the effect of the changes for you, your family, and the community you live in.

Using wearable technology, we can now easily track exercise, exertion, heart rate, and a whole set of biological variables, sharing the results with thousands of people through apps and social media accounts. There are many instances of tracking devices that live in sock drawers or where people have abused the technology by attaching them to dogs or giving them to others to wear on their behalf so as to gain extra loyalty points from health insurers. However, we all agree they are a good thing as they encourage us to move more often. As we now know, keeping active is of fundamental importance. There are also devices that monitor heart rhythm and can even alert doctors and emergency services when there is an arrhythmia. Newspapers reported that there was even a case of one of these devices being used during divorce proceedings. It was used to track the geographic location of an individual and the fact he was engaged in 'vigorous exertion' whilst in this location. In places like southern Denmark they already have a system which is up and running using drones to deliver time critical medication after a stroke. This is merely the start. Thus, wearables are going to become more important over the next few years and are also going to be incorporated within our own health records as an essential element.

The environment is changing, it is now possible to monitor activity in a home remotely using 'intelligent furniture' and the 'internet of things'. Outside, the dominance of the motor car is coming to a natural end and driverless vehicles, better open spaces, and public transport, along with cleaner air will inevitably have to happen, possibly in our lifetimes.

The effects upon our families is also going to be significant. Most people purchasing new Apple iPhones in the USA are males over the age of 65. Some say this is because they are the only people who can afford them. Older people are the most avid users of tablets and phones as this enables them to keep in touch with their families and loved ones and creates circles of care.

As we move to a new world of productive healthy ageing, the image some of us have of old age is changing. We have now started to understand the importance of retaining meaning and purpose as we grow older. Social isolation is a significant risk factor for dementia. Remaining connected with the environment and community is a sure way to help us all become more resilient. Work is also a positive factor, some of us say we should never retire, pleasing the finance ministers who want us continuing to be productive taxpayers, and there is a movement to change the name of retirement to renaissance.

There are two polarities around how to manage this significant set of changes. We can either pull the shutters up and say we want no part of it and reject it or else we can embrace it in its entirety. We suggest that you need to position yourself somewhere in the middle and, in many respects, in the future it will be easier to manage our risk factors than it is now. The emphasis needs to be on embracing rather than the rejecting the digital revolution. Whatever we choose to do, we need to remember that embracing change is part of active ageing. The image of older people as people whose world seems to get smaller and smaller is not one which aligns comfortably with the purposeful world we have tried to describe. How to achieve this in your own way and your own time and at your own pace is your responsibility of course. We will be with you on this journey, growing older but not losing the spark that made us write this book.

References

Ansari, L. (2019). *When we're 64*. Bloomsbury, London.

Bennett, D. (2019). *The New Science of Healthy Aging*. Scientific American, Springer Nature, Stuttgart.

Cavendish, C. (2019). *Extra Time*. Harper Collins, London.

Dixon, A. (2020). *The Age of Ageing Better*. Bloomsbury, London.

Gratton, L. & Scott A. (2016). *The 100-Year Life; Living and Working in the Age of Longevity*. Bloomsbury, London.

Gray, J.A.M. (2015). *Sod70!* Bloomsbury, London.

Piggott, M. (2019). *Age joyfully*. Summersdale, Chichester.

Lancet (2020). Dementia prevention, intervention, and care: 2020 report of the Lancet Commission. *Lancet*. doi:https://doi.org/10.1016/S0140-6736(20)30367-6.

Index